国家卫生和计划生育委员会"十三五"英文版规划教材
全国高等学校教材

供临床医学专业及来华留学生（MBBS）双语教学用

Epidemiology

流行病学

Raymond S. Greenberg

主　编	沈洪兵
Chief Editor	Hongbing Shen
副主编	郑志杰
Vice Chief Editor	Zhijie Zheng
	赵亚双
	Yashuang Zhao

人民卫生出版社
People's Medical Publishing House

图书在版编目（CIP）数据

流行病学：英汉对照 / 沈洪兵主编. —北京：人
民卫生出版社，2018

全国高等学校临床医学专业第一轮英文版规划教材

ISBN 978-7-117-27417-3

Ⅰ. ①流… Ⅱ. ①沈… Ⅲ. ①流行病学－高等学校－
教材－英、汉 Ⅳ. ①R18

中国版本图书馆 CIP 数据核字（2018）第 210293 号

| 人卫智网 | www.ipmph.com | 医学教育、学术、考试、健康，购书智慧智能综合服务平台 |
| 人卫官网 | www.pmph.com | 人卫官方资讯发布平台 |

流 行 病 学

主　　编：沈洪兵
出版发行：人民卫生出版社（中继线 010-59780011）
地　　址：北京市朝阳区潘家园南里 19 号
邮　　编：100021
E - mail：pmph @ pmph.com
购书热线：010-59787592　010-59787584　010-65264830
印　　刷：中国农业出版社印刷厂
经　　销：新华书店
开　　本：850×1168　1/16　印张：12
字　　数：355 千字
版　　次：2018 年 3 月第 1 版　2018 年 3 月第 1 版第 1 次印刷
标准书号：ISBN 978-7-117-27417-3
定　　价：58.00 元

打击盗版举报电话：010-59787491　E-mail：WQ @ pmph.com
（凡属印装质量问题请与本社市场营销中心联系退换）

编委（以姓氏笔画为序）

1995 年，我国首次招收全英文授课医学留学生，到 2015 年，接收临床医学专业 MBBS（Bachelor of Medicine & Bachelor of Surgery）留学生的院校达到了 40 余家，MBBS 院校数量、规模不断扩张；同时，医学院校在临床医学专业五年制、长学制教学中陆续开展不同规模和范围的双语或全英文授课，使得对一套符合我国教学实际、成体系、高质量英文教材的需求日益增长。

为了满足教学需求，进一步落实教育部《关于加强高等学校本科教学工作提高教学质量的若干意见（教高 [2001]4 号）》和《来华留学生医学本科教育（英文授课）质量控制标准暂行规定（教外来 [2007]39 号）》等相关文件的要求，规范和提高我国高等医学院校临床医学专业五年制、长学制和来华留学生（MBBS）双语教学及全英文教学的质量，推进医学双语教学和留学生教育的健康有序发展，完善和规范临床医学专业英文版教材的体系，人民卫生出版社在充分调研的基础上，于 2015 年召开了全国高等学校临床医学专业英文版规划教材的编写论证会，经过会上及会后的反复论证，最终确定组织编写一套全国规划的、适合我国高等医学院校教学实际的临床医学专业英文版教材，并计划作为 2017 年春季和秋季教材在全国出版发行。

本套英文版教材的编写结合国家卫生和计划生育委员会、教育部的总体要求，坚持"三基、五性、三特定"的原则，组织全国各大医学院校、教学医院的专家编写，主要特点如下：

1. 教材编写应教学之需启动，在全国范围进行了广泛、深入调研和论证，借鉴国内外医学人才培养模式和教材建设经验，对主要读者对象、编写模式、编写科目、编者遴选条件等进行了科学设计。

2. 坚持"三基、五性、三特定"和"多级论证"的教材编写原则，组织全国各大医学院校及教学医院有丰富英语教学经验的专家一起编写，以保证高质量出版。

3. 为保证英语表达的准确性和规范性，大部分教材以国外英文原版教科书为蓝本，根据我国教学大纲和人民卫生出版社临床医学专业第八轮规划教材主要内容进行改编，充分体现科学性、权威性、适用性和实用性。

4. 教材内部各环节合理设置，根据读者对象的特点，在英文原版教材的基础上结合需要，增加本章小结、关键术语（英中对照）、思考题、推荐阅读等模块，促进学生自主学习。

本套临床医学专业英文版规划教材共 38 种，均为国家卫生和计划生育委员会"十三五"规划教材，计划于 2017 年全部出版发行。

In 1995, China recruited overseas medical students of full English teaching for the first time. Up to 2015, more than 40 institutions enrolled overseas MBBS (Bachelor of Medicine & Bachelor of Surgery) students. The number of MBBS institutions and overseas students are continuously increasing. At the meantime, medical colleges' application for bilingual or full English teaching in different size and range in five-year and long-term professional clinical medicine teaching results to increasingly demand for a set of practical, systematic and high-qualified English teaching material.

In order to meet the teaching needs and to implement the regulations of relevant documents issued by Ministry of Education including "Some Suggestions to Strengthen the Undergraduate Teaching and to Improve the Teaching Quality" and "Interim Provisions on Quality Control Standards of International Medical Undergraduate Education (English teaching)", as well as to standardize and improve the quality of the bilingual teaching and English teaching of the five-year, long-term and international students (MBBS) of clinical medicine in China's higher medical colleges so as to promote the healthy and orderly development of medical bilingual teaching and international students education and to improve and standardize the system of English clinical medicine textbooks, after full investigation, People's Medical Publishing House (PMPH) held the writing discussion meeting of English textbook for clinical medicine department of national colleges and universities in 2015. After the repeated demonstration in and after the meeting, PMPH ultimately determined to organize the compilation of a set of national planning English textbooks which are suitable for China's actual clinical medicine teaching of medical colleges and universities. This set will be published as spring and autumn textbooks of 2017.

This set of English textbooks meets the overall requirements of the Ministry of Education and National Health and Family Planning Commission, the editorial committee includes the experts from major medical colleges and universities as well as teaching hospitals, the main features are as follows:

1. Textbooks compilation is started to meet the teaching needs, extensive and deep research and demonstration are conducted across the country, the main target readers, the model and subject of compilation and selection conditions of authors are scientifically designed in accordance with the reference of domestic and foreign medical personnel training model and experience in teaching materials.

2. Adhere to the teaching materials compiling principles of "three foundations, five characteristics, and three specialties" and "multi-level demonstration", the organization of English teaching experts with rich experience from major medical schools and teaching hospitals ensures the high quality of publication.

3. In order to ensure the accuracy and standardization of English expression, most of the textbooks are modeled on original English textbooks, and adapted based on national syllabus and main content of the eighth round of clinical medicine textbooks which were published by PMPH, fully reflecting the scientificity, authority, applicability and practicality.

4. All aspects of teaching materials are arranged reasonably, based on original textbooks,the chapter summary, key terms (English and Chinese), review questions, and recommended readings are added to promote students' independent learning in accordance with teaching needs and the characteristics of the target readers.

This set of English textbooks for clinical medicine includes 38 species which are among "13th Five-Year" planning textbooks of National Health and Family Planning Commission, and will be all published in 2017.

	教材名称		主　审	主编
28	皮肤性病学	Dermatovenereology	陈洪铎	高兴华
29	肿瘤学	Oncology		石远凯
30	眼科学	Ophthalmology		杨培增　刘奕志
31	康复医学	Rehabilitation Medicine		虞乐华
32	医学心理学	Medical Psychology		赵旭东
33	耳鼻咽喉头颈外科学	Otorhinolaryngology-Head and Neck Surgery		孔维佳
34	急诊医学	Emergency Medicine		陈玉国
35	法医学	Forensic Medicine		赵　虎
36	全球健康学	Global Health		吴群红
37	中医学	Chinese Medicine		王新华
38	医学汉语	Medical Chinese		李　骢

Preface

In pace with economic development and information globalization, internationalization has become a trend for the development and reform of higher medical education. At present, a number of medical schools in China are already offering bilingual courses in Epidemiology (including those for foreign students), mostly using self-compiled textbooks or original textbooks in English. Indeed, English textbooks are simple, straightforward, and have a close link with clinical medicine. However, their contents are not always consistent with the requirements of Epidemiology education in China. Therefore, adapting foreign textbooks to suit the actual teaching conditions in China has become the best choice.

Since its publication in 1993, *Medical Epidemiology* has been adapted for five times and translated into a number of languages. The textbook is well accepted by the international audience for its thorough explanation of key principles of Epidemiology as well as the broad range of topics it covers. Thus, the editors decided to select the third and the fifth edition of *Medical Epidemiology* as the blueprint of this rearranged version and made appropriate adaptations of its main content. The final version is composed of thirteen chapters, including the basic theories, methods and important applications of Epidemiology.

I wish to express our sincere gratitude to Mr. Raymond S. Greenberg and other editors who contributed to the original version of *Medical Epidemiology*. I would also like to acknowledge all my colleagues, who participated in the compilation of the textbook with a scientific and rigorous attitude as well as great enthusiasm. The strenuous support from People's Medical Publishing House and Nanjing Medical University is also greatly appreciated.

I hope that this textbook will help medical students in China understand more thoroughly the principles and concepts of Epidemiology. Any suggestion is heartily welcome from experts, teachers and students, in order to make this version a better one.

Hongbing Shen
Nanjing, China

Contents

Introduction to Epidemiology

PATIENTS PROFILE

A 29-year-old previously healthy man was referred to the University of California at Los Angeles (UCLA) Medical Center with a history of fever, fatigue, lymph node enlargement, and weight loss of almost 25 lb over the preceding 8 months. He had a temperature of 39.5℃ appeared physically wasted, and had swollen lymph nodes. Laboratory evaluation revealed a depressed level of peripheral blood lymphocytes. The patient suffered from simultaneous infections involving Candida albicans in his upper digestive tract, cytomegalovirus in his urinary tract, and Pneumocystis carinii in his lungs. Although antibiotic therapy was administered, the patient remained severely ill.

INTRODUCTION

Epidemiology is the study of the distribution and determinants of health-related states or events in specified populations, and the application of this study to the control of health problems. Specifically, epidemiologists examine patterns of illness in the population and then try to determine why certain groups or individuals develop a particular disease whereas others do not.

Knowledge about who is likely to develop a particular disease and under what circumstances they are likely to develop it is central to the daily practice of medicine and to efforts to improve the health of the public. To prevent an illness, health care providers must be able both to identify persons who, because of personal characteristics or their environment, are at high risk and to intervene to reduce that risk. This type of knowledge emerges in many cases from epidemiologic research.

This book serves as an introduction to epidemiologic methods and the way in which these methods can be used to answer key medical and public health questions. This chapter begins by considering a single disease, as described in the Patient Profile. Focusing attention on one disease enables us to demonstrate the important contribution of epidemiology to current knowledge about this condition. Although the emphasis is on a single disease, it should be recognized that epidemiologic methods can be applied to wide spectrum of conditions ranging from acute illness, such as outbreaks of food-borne infections, to long-term debilitating conditions, such as Alzheimer's disease.

The man in the Patient Profile was referred to the UCLA Medical Center in June 1981. At the time, there was no obvious explanation as to why a healthy young man would suddenly develop concurrent infections in three different organ systems involving three different microorganisms. More surprising was the nature of the infections that were present. Opportunistic infections, such as those caused by the parasite P. carinii, are infectious illnesses, that tend to occur only in persons with lowered resistance as may result from impaired immune response. The young man described in the Patient Profile; however, did not have any obvious underlying causes of immune dysfunction. For example, he did not have cancer or severe malnutrition and he did not use immune-suppressing drugs. Why then was his body overwhelmed by the infections? This question was given a heightened sense of urgency by the severity of the patient's illness.

This patient was not the first to be referred to the UCLA Medical Center with this clinical presentation.

Within the preceding 6 months three other previously healthy young men with recent histories of weight loss, fever, and lymph node enlargement had been examined. All had P carinii pneumonia and C albicans infections.

Why were four patients with similar symptoms appearing at about the same time in the same location? Suspecting that the illnesses in these four patients might be related, the UCLA physicians notified pubic health officials and prepared a descriptive report of their findings for publication.

Was this new appearance of a rare and life-threatening form of pneumonia confined to the UCAL Medical Center or was it being observed by physicians elsewhere? If the experience at UCLA was unique, the entire episode might be regarded as a medical curiosity---unusual, but not a reason for great public health concern. On the other hand, if patients similar to those at UCLA were appearing in clinics or medical offices elsewhere, this episode could not be easily dismissed. Within a matter of weeks, public health authorities received reports of outbreaks of P carinii pneumonia among previously healthy young men in San Francisco and New York City.

In the United States, the federal agency that is responsible for monitoring unusual patents of disease occur is the Centers for Disease Control and Prevention (CDC). Recognizing the potential for the widespread emergence of this new, unexplained, and debilitating condition, the CDC established a special task force to collect more detailed information on the affected persons. In addition, the CDC issued a formal request to report such patients to all state health departments. Between June and November 1981, 76 instances of P.carinii pneumonia were identified in persons who did not have known predisposing illnesses and were not taking immune-suppressing medications. A few months later, the disease that afflicted these patients was named the acquired immune deficiency syndrome (AIDS).

PERSON, PLACE, & TIME

The physicians at UCLA played a crucial role in establishing the presence of a new disease in their community. The first few affected patients identified with any outbreak of disease are referred to as sentinel case. The story of the first few AIDS patients is particularly dramatic because of the severity of the illness and the extent and speed with which the disease spread to others. A sudden and great increase in the occurrence of a disease within a community or region of a disease (or other health-related condition) that is clearly in excess of normal expectancy is referred to as an **epidemic.** It quickly became apparent; however, that the emergence of AIDS was not confined to a few communities. A rapidly emerging outbreak of disease that affects a wide range of geographically distributed populations is described as a **pandemic.** In 1981, no one could have predicted that by 1998 almost 650,000 persons in the USA would be diagnosed with AIDS and almost 400,000 deaths from AIDS would be reported nationally. By 1996, AIDS was the eighth most common cause of death in the USA and the third most common cause of death for persons between the age 25 and 44 years. With the introduction of effective combination drug therapy, the death rate from AIDS has declined in the USA and in other industrialized nations. In developing nations a much more devastating picture is emerging; for instance, in sub-Saharan Africa, it is estimated that over 7% of young adults have AIDS.

Looking back to 1981, when AIDS was not yet recognized as a clinical entity, it is instructive to consider the features of the sentinel cases that suggested a possible connection. All the patients with AIDS who presented to the UCLA clinicians suffered from the same rare opportunistic infections. Had the infections involved more conventional human pathogens-or less severe symptoms---the entire episode might have gone unnoticed for some time.

Beyond their clinical similarities, the sentinel cases shared other features, as summarized in Table 1-1. All four patients were previously healthy homosexual men in their early 30s (personal characteristics) who resided in Los Angeles (place) and first became ill in the 9 months ending in June 1981(time). These three dimensions---persons, place, and time---are the features traditionally used to characterize patterns of disease occurrence or descriptive epidemiology, as discussed in Chapter 4.

Table 1-1 Characteristics of sentinel cases of AIDS in Los Angeles, 1981

Characteristics of Sentinel Cases	Personal Attributes
Age	Early 30s
Gender	Male
Prior health	Good
Sexual preference	Homosexual
Place of occurrence	Los Angeles
Time of occurrence	October 19, 1980 to June 19, 1981

THE EPIDEMIOLOGIC APPROACH

Epidemiology is concerned with the distribution and determinants of disease frequency in population. Interest in frequency or occurrence of disease derives largely from a basic tenet of epidemiology, ie, **disease does not develop at random**. In essence, all persons are not equally likely to develop a particular disease. The level of risk for different individuals typically is a function of their personal characteristics and environment. The characterization of a disease pattern by personal characteristics such as age, race, and sex, environmental factors and behaviors is one of the fundamental applications of epidemiology. It is what one might refer to as a **descriptive use** and serves a vital purpose in helping to identify high-risk individuals within the population. In addition to the descriptive role of epidemiology, another application referred to as **analytic**. In this context, epidemiologic methods are used to understand the determinants, or causes of disease.

As applied to the outbreak of AIDS, for instance, it is highly unlikely that of the first four cases in Los Angeles each would have occurred in homosexual males if the disease was striking at random. The repeated occurrence of AIDS in homosexual men suggested that this segment of the population had an increased risk of developing the disease. Other high-risk groups for AIDS, including hemophiliacs and injecting drug users, were soon identified. On the surface, these three groups seemed to have little in common. On closer examination, however, it became evident that an increased risk of exposure to the blood of other persons was the factor they all share. Contemporary medical research is devoted largely to investigating the biologic elements of disease development. For example, in the study of AIDS, a microbiologist tends to focus on the infectious agent, human immunodeficiency virus (HIV). An immunologist might concentrate on the primary target of HIV infection, the $CD4^+T$ lymphocyte, which coordinates a number of immune functions. The epidemiologist, on the other hand, views a disease from both a biologic and a social perspective. It is not enough to know that HIV is transmitted primary through contaminated blood. The epidemiologist must be able to understand the circumstances of HIV transmission among humans. Here, the influence of social factors is undeniable. The spread of AIDS in human populations cannot be fully appreciated without recognizing the role of certain behaviors, such as sexual practices or injecting drug use.

The desire to study social factors that impinge on health has definite implications for how epidemiologic research is conducted. In most instances, this research involves observations of phenomena that occur naturally within human populations. Such an approach is unique among the medical sciences. Two features distinguish the epidemiologic approach from other biomedical sciences: (1) the focus on human populations and (2) a heavy reliance on nonexperimental observations.

At first, the focus on human populations may not seem distinctive. Ultimately, all medical research is motivated by a desire to prevent or control human illnesses. The process leading to that goal, however, may take various routes. Laboratory scientists, for example, often rely on experiments that involve nonhuman animals, cells in tissue culture, or biochemical assays. Although these studies offer important advantages to the investigators, such as precise control over the experimental conditions, certain limitations must also be recognized. Obviously, a laboratory environment may not accurately reflect the actual conditions of exposure in the external world. Of equal importance is the recognition that animals of different species may have dissimilar responses to experimental manipulations. It cannot be assumed that biological effects detected in rodents will necessarily apply to humans.

Epidemiologists avoid these concerns by attempting to study people directly in their natural environments. With this approach, it is not necessary to make assumptions about similarity of effects either across species or across doses and routes of exposure. The epidemiologist actually observes the patterns of exposure and disease development as they naturally occur within human populations. Without such information, it would not be possible to reach a definitive conclusion about the extent of disease related to a particular agent.

As with any scientific method, the epidemiologic approach has inherent constraints. In observational research, which comprises much of epidemiology, the investigator merely watches the phenomena under study, ie, the epidemiologist has no control over the events that occur. It is often difficult, therefore, to separate the causal contributions of the exposure of interest from the causal contributions of other background influences in the population. Even direct measurement of the degree of exposure may not be possible in some settings, thereby forcing the epidemiologist to rely on indirect estimates.

The epidemiologist's perspective of the relationship between exposure to risk factors and the development of disease in human populations may appear rather crude in comparison to the exacting research performed at the molecular level. The epidemiologist frequently sees only how different levels of exposure across groups of the population affect the comparative likelihood that those groups will develop disease. Typically, the epidemiologist can identify the personal, social, and environmental circumstances under which a disease tends to occur, without being able to explain the exact processes that give rise to the disease. In traditional epidemiology, it was treated as a "black box." However, with the development of **molecular epidemiology**, the epidemiologist assesses the biologic basis of an association by using biologic measurements to assess biomark-

ers. In this way, the epidemiologist may help open up the "black box" by examining the events intermediate between exposure and disease occurrence or progression. Medical progress often is best advanced when the sciences that focus on subcellular and molecular basic research work in tandem with the population-oriented science of epidemiology. For example, as bench scientists were struggling to characterize the molecular properties of HIV, epidemiologist already determined that AIDS is a contagious disease that is spread through certain interpersonal behaviors. As the painstaking search continues for improved treatment, or even a cure or vaccine, public health professionals have recommended measures to prevent the spread of HIV by reducing the frequency of the following high-risk practices: (1) causal, unprotected sex and (2) sharing needles among injecting drug user. Furthermore, the application of molecular epidemiology has greatly improved the ability to analyze the origin of HIV and track the spread of this pathogen.

THE APPLICATIONS OF EPIDEMIOLOGY

Epidemiologic methods can be used for a number of distinct purposes. In the following sections, these areas of application are specified, with corresponding illustrations drawn from the literature on AIDS.

DISEASE SURVEILLANCE

Perhaps the most basic question that can be asked about a disease is "what is the frequency with which the disease occur?" To answer this question, it is necessary to know the number of persons who acquire the disease (cases) over a specified period of time and the size of the unaffected population. Typically, the criteria used to define the occurrence of a disease depend on current knowledge about the disease; such criteria may become more refined as the causes of a disease are delineated and new diagnostic tests are introduced. For example, in 1982, the CDC created an initial, relatively simple surveillance definition for AIDS:

A disease, at least moderately indicative of a defect in cell-mediated immunity, occurring in a person with no known cause for diminished resistance to that disease.

A more specific definition became possible once the causative agent, HIV, was identified and tests for the detection of antibodies to the virus were developed. In 1987, the CDC surveillance definition was expanded to incorporate clinical conditions that are indicative of AIDS. A 1993 revision further expanded the surveillance definition to include three additional indicator conditions (pulmonary tuberculosis, recurrent pneumonia, or invasive cervical cancer) or the presence of a severely depressed $CD4^+$ T-lymphocyte count.

In the USA, a number of diseases, including AIDS, must be reported to public health authorities. Monitoring the patterns of occurrence of a disease within a population is referred to as **surveillance**. Public health surveillance is a long-term, continuous and systematic process of collection, analysis, interpretation, and dissemination of data on dynamic trends of disease and of factors that influence disease incidence. Results of analyses of disease surveillance data are reported to the individuals and organizations that are responsible for preventing and controlling disease so that they can intervene in a timely manner and evaluate the effects of their programs. There are many potential benefits from the collection of surveillance data. This type of information (1) can help to identify the new outbreak of illness, such as AIDS, (2) can provide clues, by considering the population groups that are most affected by the illness, to possible causes of the condition ,(3) can be used to suggest strategies to control or prevent the spread of disease, (4) can be used to measure the impact of disease prevention and control efforts and finally, (5) can provide information on the burden of illness, necessary for determining health and medical service needs.

For surveillance purposes, the size of the source population from which cases arise usually is estimated from census data. The frequency of disease occurrence is then expressed as the number of new cases developing within a specified time among a standard number of unaffected individuals. For example, during 1997 over 60,000 cases of AIDS were reported in the USA; the U.S. population in 1997 was almost 270,000,000. Dividing the number

of reported case by the size of the population yields 0.00022 cases per person during that year. For ease of communication, epidemiologists typically express such frequencies of disease occurrence for a population of a specified size, say 100,000 persons. By multiplying 0.00022 by 100,000, the number 22 is obtained. That is to say, within a standard population of 100,000 persons in the U.S. 22 persons would have been reported as developing AIDS during 1997. This measure of the rapidity of disease occurrence is referred to as an **incidence rate**. More information on incidence rates is presented in Chapter 2.

SEARCHING FOR CAUSES

To study personal and environmental characteristics, epidemiologists often rely on interviews, review of records, and laboratory examinations. Though such sources of information, a profile of characteristics that accompany the disease can be generated. Associations between these characteristics and the occurrence of disease can arise by coincidence, by noncausal linkages to other features, or by cause-and-effect relationships. Of course, the epidemiologist is primarily interested in the last category, ie, determinants of disease development, also known as **risk factors**. Identification of risk factors can result in a better understanding of the pathways leading to disease acquisition and, consequently, better strategies for prevention.

Again, returning to the AIDS example, early epidemiologic studies played an important role in determining the cause of this disease. Within the first 5 months after recognition of this syndrome, the CDC had received reports on 70 patients with AIDS in four urban centers. Of these individuals, 50 homosexual male patients with AIDS were interviewed; also interviewed were 120 unaffected homosexual male comparison subjects. Persons who are affected with a disease are referred to by epidemiologists as **cases**, and unaffected comparison persons are called **controls**. Comparisons of the responses from cases and controls revealed that the AIDS patients had a higher number of sexual partners. This type of investigation is referred to as a **case-control study**; the basic design of such a study is illustrated Figure 1-1.

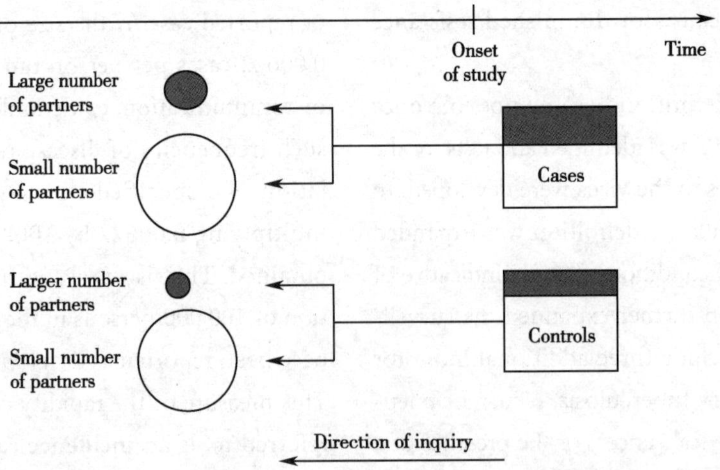

Onset
of study

Time

Large number
of partners

Small number
of partners

Cases

Larger number
of partners

Small number
of partners

Controls

Direction of inquiry

Figure 1-1. Schematic diagram of a case-control study of the association between the number of male sexual partners of homosexual men and the risk of AIDS. Shaded areas represent subjects with a large number of sexual partners and unshaded areas represent subjects with a small number of sexual partners.

In essence, this study is an attempt to look backward in time to identify characteristics that may have contributed to the development of the disease. The increased number of sexual partners---as well as a greater frequency of syphilis among cases---suggested that AIDS resulted from a sexually transmitted infectious agent, later discovered to be the HIV virus. Case-control studies are described in Chapter 6.

Comparison of historical exposures reported by cases and controls can provide suggestive evidence of a cause-and-effect relationship. This type of information, however, may be distorted or **biased** by the fact that the ability of cases and controls to recall earlier exposure differs. Such bias could be avoided by using a **cohort study** design in which exposure is assessed among unaffected persons, and subjects are then observed for subsequent development of illness. To collect such data, a cohort of 2507 homosexual men without antibodies to HIV (seronegative) was questioned about their sexual practices and then followed for development of antibodies to HIV (seroconversion). Within 6 months, 95 men (3.8%) seroconverted, and the likelihood or **risk** of developing HIV antibodies was found to be related to receptive anal intercourse. The basic design of this cohort study is illustrated schematically in Figure 1-2. Cohort studies are discussed in Chapter 5.

DIAGNOSTIC TESTING

The purpose of diagnostic testing is to obtain objective evidence of the presence or absence of a particular condition. This evidence can be obtained to detect

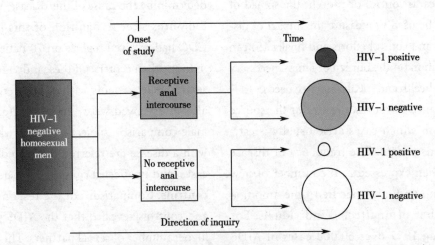

Onset
of study

Time

HIV–1 positive

Receptive
anal
intercourse

HIV–1 negative

HIV–1
negative
homosexual
men

HIV–1 positive

No receptive
anal
intercourse

HIV–1 negative

Direction of inquiry

Figure 1-2. Schematic diagram of a cohort study of the association between receptive anal intercourse and risk of being HIV positive. Shaded areas indicate subjects who practice receptive anal intercourse and unshaded areas represent subjects who do not.

disease as its earliest stages among asymptomatic persons in the general population, a process referred to as **screening.** In other circumstances, diagnostic tests are used to confirm a diagnosis among persons with existing signs or symptoms of illness. Ideally, a diagnostic test would correctly distinguish affected persons from unaffected persons; unfortunately, as is true of most diagnostic tests, assays for HIV infection are not perfect.

Occasionally, a positive test result will incorrectly suggest that infection is present in an unaffected person. This type of outcome is referred to as a **false positive**, because the positive test result was in error. Obviously, a false-positive finding for HIV infection could be devastating to the tested individual, so every effort must be made to keep such errors to a minimum. A test with a very low percentage of false-positive results is said to have high **specificity** (see Figure 1-3).

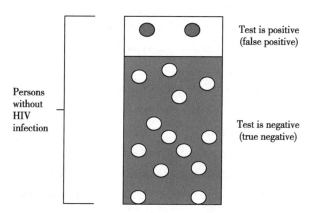

Figure 1-3. When a diagnostic test is applied to persons without HIV infection, it is highly specific if the true negative test results (shaded area) greatly outnumber erroneous positive test results (unshaded area).

Another type of error occurs when a test incorrectly suggests that infection is not present (negative test result) in an affected person. This type of outcome is referred to as a **false negative**, because the negative test result was in error. A false-negative finding for HIV infection could provide inappropriate reassurance to an infected person, thereby delaying the start of treatment and perhaps increasing the risk of spread to other persons. A test with a very low percentage of false-negative results is described as having high **sensitivity** (see Figure 1-4). More detail on measures of test accuracy is presented in Chapter 8.

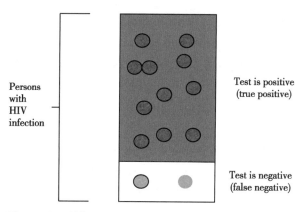

Figure 1-4. When a diagnostic test is applied to persons with HIV infection, it is highly sensitive if the true positive test results (shaded area) greatly outnumber erroneous negative test results (unshaded area).

A number of different tests for the presence of HIV infection are available. The screening approach used most widely is to attempt to detect antibodies to the virus. This strategy is based on two assumptions: (1) HIV-infected persons have detectable antibodies and (2) persons with detectable antibodies to the virus are infected with HIV. In practice, these assumptions appear to be reasonably valid among patients beyond the first few months of infection. The time required to mount an antibody response sufficient for detection (seroconversion) varies across patients, but the vast majority seroconvert in less than 6 months following initial HIV infection.

The performance of an enzyme-linked immunosorbent assay (ELISA) test for antibodies to HIV was first reported in 1985. Among 74 patients who met the CDC clinical surveillance definition for AIDS and had unequivocal ELISA test results, 72(97%) had detectable antibodies. In other words, a false-negative outcome was observed for only 2 patients(2%). Among 261 healthy blood donors with unequivocal ELISA test results, 257(98%) had no detectable antibodies (ie, a false-positive outcome was found for 4 persons [2%]). Thus, the ELISA test was judged to be both sensitive and specific, and it has become the most widely employed screening test for HIV infection.

Considering the potential for error, it is recommended that a positive ELISA test be repeated in duplicate. If either of the following-up tests is positive, a supplementary test should be performed. The most widely used confirmatory test is the Western blot. This type of test is not recommended for screening purposes, because Western blot can produce a substantial proportion of equivocal results among persons who are negative to all other HIV tests. Additionally, the presence of infection with HIV can be detected through other approaches, such as the detection of an antigen of the virus, p24, in the serum or the plasma of infected patients, and the polymerase chain reaction (PCR) to amplify viral genetic material so that HIV can be detected in minute concentrations.

DETERMINING THE NATURE HISTORY

After being informed of a new diagnosis, patients most frequently ask "what will happen to me?" This question cannot be answered with certainty because of variations in outcome among individuals. Consider, for example, a patient newly diagnosed as being HIV positive. In this instance, with the advent of new treatments it is reasonable to questions whether the full syndrome of AIDS will develop and if it does how long it will take to occur. In attempting to address these questions, the physician might consult published research on the progression of HIV-related illness. Usually these data are collected on large groups of patients. By noting the timing of critical events for each patient (eg, date of determination of HIV infection, development of clinical symptoms of illness, demonstrable changes in immune function, diagnosis of AIDS, and subsequent clinical events), the progression of the disease can be divided into phases.

When these events are summarized for many patients, precise and accurate estimates of the typical sequence of events---the **nature history** of the illness---can be constructed. Some authors restrict the use of the descriptor "nature" to situations in which medical treatment is unavailable or ineffective. Others use the term more broadly to indicate the typical course of an illness, regardless of whether it can be treated effectively.

There are several ways to characterize the natural history of an illness. One straightforward measure is the **case fatality**, which represents the percentage of patients with a disease who die within a specified observation period. For example, among 11,740 reported adolescent and adult patients diagnosed with AIDS in 1985 in the USA, 10,946 are known to have died before 1998. In other words, the case fatality was

$$10,946/11\,740 \times 100\% = 93.2\%$$

The approach to determining the case fatality is illustrated schematically in Figure 1-5.

Another method of characterizing the nature history of a disease is to estimate the typical duration from diagnosis to death (**survival time**). As an illustration, a study was conducted in a rural part of Uganda, a country in which 8% of adults are infected with HIV. In this setting, in which economic and other conditions limited treatment to simple and affordable drugs, the nature history of HIV infection was characterized. The study involved persons who were seropositive for HIV and a compari-

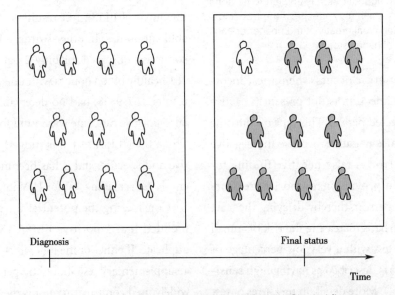

Figure 1-5. Schematic diagram of the concept of case fatality. Shaded figure represented patients who are deceased and unshaded figures represent patients who are alive.

son group of seronegative individuals. All subjects were identified in 1990 and were evaluated clinically every 3 months until death or the end of calendar year 1995, whichever came first. For the initial 3 years after seroconversion, there was no difference in survival between the HIV-positive persons and the persons without infection. By 5 years following seroconversion, however, only 83% of the HIV-positive persons were still alive, compared with 94% of the seronegative persons.

A number of factors can affect the apparent nature history of HIV related illness. HIV infection may exist for a prolonged period of time prior to the development of symptoms that lead to a clinical diagnosis of AIDS. Recognition of the presence of infection during this preclinical phase clearly depends on the availability of an effective screening test, the sensitivity of the test to detect early infection, and the extent to which the screening test is applied in the population. The expectation, therefore, is that in the earliest years of the AIDS epidemic, prior to the development and widespread application of screening tests for HIV, the diagnosis was made at comparatively advanced stages of infection, when symptoms already were evident.

Changes over time in the criteria used to diagnose AIDS could also alter the apparent survival experience of patients with this disease. For example, analysis of patients with HIV registered in Italy between July 1987 and December 1991 revealed that when the 1987 CDC case definition for AIDS was applied, half of the patients survived for 24 months more or longer. The length of survival that is met or exceeded by 50% of the study population is referred to as the **median survival time**. When the broadened 1993 CDC case definition was retrospectively applied to this same population, not only did a larger number of patients meet the definition, but the median survival time was found to exceed 57 months. In other words, the population of patients who met the 1993 case definition tended to have a more favorable outcome than the subset that met the earlier definition.

SEARCHING FOR PROGNOSTIC FACTORS

Analysis of survival can be employed to identify groups of patients with unusually favorable (or unfavorable) clinical outcomes. Characteristics that relate to the likelihood of survival are referred to as **prognostic factors**. The approach to identifying prognostic factors can be illustrated by a study conducted by Mellors and colleagues (1997). Using data collected from the Multicenter AIDS Cohort Study of homosexual men in the USA, the investigators evaluated factors related to the progression from initial infection with HIV to two clinical end points: (1) the development of AIDS and (2) AIDS-related death. A total of 1604 men enrolled in the study, which include a follow-up period on average of almost 10 years. Over this time period, 998 of the participants developed AIDS and 855 died of AIDS. The design of this study is depicted schematically in Figure 1-6. Figure 1-6 shows that the study design is similar to that of cohort study (Figure 1-2), except

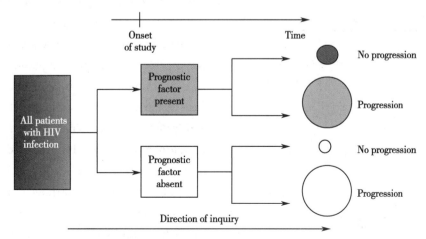

Figure 1-6. Schematic diagram of a study to evaluate prognostic factors for persons with HIV infection. The shaded areas represent patients with the favorable prognostic factor of interest and unshaded areas represent. without the favorable prognostic factor of interest.

that the focus is on predicting survival rather than on determining risk factors for the onset of disease.

In the study by Mellors et al, a number of potential prognostic factors were assessed, including, among other, oral candidiasis or fever, markers of immune stimulation, various lymphocyte counts, including CD4+T-lymphocytes, and an assay of the plasma concentration of HIV-1 RNA (ribonucleic acid---the genetic material of the virus). The HIV-1 RNA assay provides a precise measurement of the load of the virus circulating in a patient's blood. As might be expected, some association was seen between the initial levels of the individual prognostic factors. For example, patients with higher virus loads at the start of the study were more likely to have fever or oral candidiasis and reduced levels of CD4+T-lymphocyte levels. Virus load also was seen as the single best predictor of the subsequent decline over time in CD4+T-lymphocyte levels as well as in the progression to AIDS and the death. Specifically, when study subjects were grouped into five ordered categories based on plasma virus load, the 6-year probability of AIDS-related death ranged from 1% among those with the lightest load to 70% among those with the heaviest load. By combining information of HIV-1 RNA concentrations with CD4+T-lymphocyte levels, even more effective determination of the likelihood of disease progression could be made. The results of this investigation established plasma HIV-1 RNA as the preferred clinical marker for monitoring the status of HIV infection and for assessing prognosis (Table 1-2).

Table 1-2 Independent prognostic factors for AIDS

Factors	Poor prognosis level
Age	37 years or old
Initial presentation	Multiple diagnoses
Single diagnosis other than Kaposi's sarcoma or P carinii Pneumonia	Thrush
CD4+T-lymphocytes	Low
Hemogolobin	Low

TESTING NEW TREATMENT

All new medications must be tested and proved effective before they can be introduced into routine clinical care. The standard approach used to evaluate treatment effectiveness is the **randomized controlled trials**. The term "controlled" means that patients (experimental subjects) who receive the new medication are compared with patients (control subjects) who receive either an inactive substance (placebo) or a standard treatment if one exists. "Randomized" refers to a method of assignment of subjects to ether the experimental or control group that is determined by chance rather than patient preference or physician selection. This type of allocation system is desirable because it tend to result in study groups that are comparable with respect to important prognostic factors. Randomized controlled clinical trials are discussed in Chapter 7.

The principles of randomized controlled clinical trials can be demonstrated by a study that has contributed to a revolution in the treatment of HIV-infected persons. That study, published by Hammer and colleagues in 1997, compared a standard therapy with a new experimental treatment regimen. The standard therapy employed two drugs (zidovudine and lamivudine), both of which are inhibitors of the HIV reverse transcriptase. By interfering with the conversion of viral genetic material to a form that can be incorporated into the host, these drugs limit the replication of HIV within host cells. The experimental treatment involved these two drugs plus another one (indinavir), which is an inhibitor of the HIV protease. Protease inhibitors interfere with the process of assembling viral components after replication of HIV genetic material. The experimental therapy, therefore, involved a simultaneous attack on two separate and distinct steps in the process of HIV reproduction. Prior studies had demonstrated that this combined therapy was capable of reducing viral plasma load and raising CD4+T-lymphocyte levels. Since favorable responses were seen in these prognostic factors, it was reasonable to anticipate that this combination therapy might diminish the rate of progression of HIV-related disease.

Hammer and colleagues undertook a randomized controlled clinical trial in which a standard two-drug reverse transcriptase regimen was compared with a three-drug combined reverse transcriptase/protease inhibition experimental treatment. The basic design of the trial is depicted in Figure 1-7. Participants were

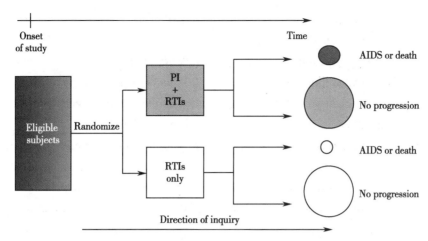

Figure 1-7. Schematic diagram of a randomized controlled clinical trial of reverse transcriptase inhibitors (RTIs), with or without a protease inhibitor (PI), for the treatment of HIV infection. The shaded area indicates patients randomized to receive combined treatment with RTIs and a PI.

recruited from 40 different clinical centers throughout the USA. The subjects were required to have documentation of HIV infection and a $CD4^+$T-lymphocyte level diminished below a predetermined level. To minimized effects of prior therapy, eligible subjects were limited to those who had not been treated previously with a protease inhibitors. A total of 1156 patients were randomized between January 1997, with 579 assigned to the standard therapy group and the remaining 577 assigned to the experimental therapy group. The clinical characteristics of the two groups were similar at the onset of treatment. After an average of about 38 weeks of observation, the trial was terminated because of a dramatic difference in risk of disease progression between the two groups. Within the experimental treatment group of the study, 33 patients (6%) progressed to AIDS or died. In contrast, within the standard treatment group, 63 patients (11%) progressed to AIDS or died.

The results of this trial and other similar studies clearly demonstrated the short-term therapeutic benefit of combined treatment with reverse transcriptase inhibitors and protease inhibitors. The ethical imperative to terminate this study early because of the substantial advantage of combination therapy left unresolved the question of whether this effect is sustainable over longer periods of time. Even without data on the long-term benefits, the striking results of the studies of combined reverse transcriptase and protease inhibition changed the whole approach to

clinical management of HIV infection. As the search for even more effective treatments continues, randomized controlled clinical trials will serve as the definitive approach to establishing therapeutic superiority.

SUMMARY

In this chapter, we have seen how epidemiologic search has contributed to basic knowledge about AIDS.

(1) The techniques of surveillance were used to determine the patterns of HIV infection and occurrence of AIDS by person, place, and time.

(2) Comparisons of affected and unaffected persons led to the identification of risk factors and ultimately to the suspicion that an infectious agent was responsible for the disease.

(3) Evaluation of tests for antibodies to HIV allowed improved diagnosis and prevention of spread by contaminated blood products.

(4) Studies of natural history helped to define the clinical course of the illness.

(5) Prognostic factors were determined through comparison of patients with favorable outcomes.

(6) Finally, improvement in treatment was demonstrated through randomized controlled clinical trials.

The story of HIV and AIDS is particularly dramatic because it involves a devastating disease that emerged rapidly in the population and developed with minimal advance warning. It is an unfinished story because new cases are still occurring with alarming frequency, and a cure has not yet been identified. Epidemiology will continue to play an important role in monitoring progress in the prevention and treatment of HIV-related illness and AIDS.

Epidemiologic research has been pivotal in gaining insight into many different diseases. From infectious illnesses to heart disease to cancer to congenital malformations, epidemiology has provided insight into patterns of disease occurrence and underlying causal factors. Ultimately, this information can be used to help control the impact of disease either through preventive measures or improved clinical management.

(Hongbing Shen)

IMPORTANT TERMINOLOGY

epidemiology	流行病学
epidemic	流行
pandemic	大流行
molecular epidemiology	分子流行病学
disease surveillance	疾病监测
risk factors	危险因素
case-control study	病例对照研究
cohort study	队列研究
risk	发病风险
screening	筛查
false positive	假阳性
false negative	假阴性
specificity	特异度
sensitivity	灵敏度
nature history	自然史
case fatality	病死率
survival time	生存时间
median survival time	中位生存时间
prognostic factors	预后因子
randomized controlled clinical trial	随机对照试验

 STUDY QUESTIONS

Questions 1-8: For each numbered situation below, select the most appropriate term from the following lettered options. Each option can be used once, more than once, or not at all.

A. *Epidemic*   B. *Incidence rate*

C. *Risk*   D. *Sensitivity*

E. *Specificity*   F. *Case fatality*

G. *Risk factor*   H. *Prognostic factor*

1. *What is the best descriptor of the likelihood over 10 years that an initially unaffected person will develop hypertension?*

2. *What the best descriptor of a characteristic, such as hypertension, that affects the likelihood of developing a new myocardial infarction?*

3. *What is the best descriptor of the rapidity with which new cases of myocardial infarction occur among a population of previously unaffected persons?*

4. *What is the best descriptor of the percentage of persons unaffected by an acute myocardial infarction who are classified correctly by a diagnostic test, such as a cardiac troponin T assay?*

5. *What is the best descriptor of a characteristic, such as the severity of coronary artery blockage, that affects the duration of survival following an acute myocardial infarction?*

6. *What is the best descriptor of a sudden unexpected rise in the frequency of occurrence of acute myocardial infarction in a community?*

7. *What is the best descriptor of the percentage of patients with a acute myocardial infarction who die within 10 years of the their initial diagnosis?*

8. *What is the best descriptor of the percentage of persons with an acute myocardial infarction who are classified correctly by a diagnostic test, such as a cardiac troponin t assay?*

Question 9-13: For each measure described in the numbered statements below, select the most appropriate numerical value from the following lettered options. Each option can be used once, more than once, or none at all.

A. *0.02*   B. *1.0*

C. *1.6*   D. *2.0*

E. *5.0*   F. *20*

G. *80*   H. *90*

9. *What is the annual incidence rate (per 1000 persons) of colon cancer, if it is diagnosed in 1 person year within a community of 500 unaffected individuals, assuming that one-fifth of the affected individuals die from the condition?*

10. *What is the 5-year cumulative risk (in %) of developing colon cancer in the community described in question 9, assuming there are no migrations into or out of the community and no deaths from other cause?*

11. *What is the case fatality (in %) of colon cancer in the community described question 9?*

12. *A screening test is applied to residents of the community described in question 9. What is the sensitivity (in %) of the screening test if it detects 8 of 10 persons with colon cancer and correctly determines that 405 unaffected persons do not have colon cancer?*

13. *What is the specificity (in %) of the screening test described in the question 12?*

FURTHER READING

Overview of Epidemiology

Raymond S. Greenberg: Medical Epidemiology (3rd edition). The McGraw-Hill Companies, Inc. 2001.

Overview of AIDS

Horowitz HW et al: Human immunodeficiency virus infection, Part I. Disease-A-Month. 1998;44:545.

REFERENCES

Patient Profile

Gottlieb MS ,et al.Pneumocystis carinii pneumonia and mucosal candidiasis in previously healthy homosexual men: evidence of a new acquired cellular immunodeficiency. *N Engl J Med.* 1981;305:1425.

Person, Place and Time

CDC: HIV/AIDS Surveillance Report 1997;9(No.2):1.

Disease Surveillance

CDC: 1993 revised classification system for HIV infection and expanded surveillance case definition for AIDS among adolescents and adults. *MMWR.* 1992;41(RR-17):1.

CDC:HIV/AIDS Surveillance Report 1997;9(No.2):1.

Fleming PL, et al.Declines in AIDS incidence and deaths in the USA: a signal change in the epidemic. *AIDS.* 1998;12 (Suppl A):555.

Searching for Causes

de Vincenzi I. European Study Group on Heterosexual Transmission of HIV: A longitudinal study of human immunodeficiency virus transmission by heterosexual partners. *N Engl J Med.* 1994;331:341.

Jaffe HW, et al. National case-control study of Kaposi's sarcoma and Pneumocystis carinii pneumonia in homosexual men: Part 1. Epidemiologic results. *Ann Intern Med.* 1983;99:145.

Kingsley LA, et al. Risk factors for seroconversion to human immunodeficiency virus among male homosexuals. *Lancet.* 1987;1:345.

Lemp GF ,et al. Seroprevalence of HIV and risk behaviors among young homosexual and bisexual men. *JAMA.* 1994;272:449.

Diagnostic Testing

Phair JP, Wolinsky S.Diagnosis of infection with the human immunodeficiency virus. *Clin Infect Dis.* 1992;15:13.

Proffitt MR, Yen-Lieberman B. Laboratory diagnosis of human immunodeficiency virus infection. *Infect Dis Clin North Am.* 1993;7:203.

Weiss SH et al: Screening test for HTLV-Ⅲ (AIDS agent) antibodies. *JAMA.* 1985;253:221.

Determining the Natural History

CDC:HIV/AIDS Surveillance Report 1997;9(No.2):19.

Morgan D,et al. An HIV-1 natural history cohort and survival times in rural Uganda. *AIDS.* 1997;11:633.

Vella S, et al. Differential survival of patients with AIDS according to the 1987 and 1993 CDC case definitions. *JAMA.* 1994;271:1197.

Searching for Prognostic Factors

Mellors JW.Plasma viral load and CD4[+] lymphocytes as prognostic markers of HIV-1 infection. *Ann Intern Med.* 1997;126:946.

Testing New Treatments

Hammer SM, et al. A controlled trial of two nucleoside analogues plus indinavir in persons with human immunodeficiency virus infection and CD4 cell counts of 200 per cubic millimeter or less. *N Engl J Med.* 1997;337:725.

Epidemiologic Measures

HEALTH SCENARIO

Mr. W., a 73-year-old retired insurance executive, presented to the emergency department of his local hospital with a recent onset of shortness of breath and chest pain when breathing. The patient had undergone a total hip replacement (arthroplasty) 7 days earlier at the same hospital. He had been discharged on postoperative day 4 and was encouraged to ambulate as much as possible at home while recovering. His mobility was limited, however, because of pain on standing, and he had not yet begun a prescribed physical therapy regimen. Mr. W. was a 40-pack-year cigarette smoker and was morbidly obese.

Upon physical examination, the patient appeared anxious and was breathing rapidly (respiratory rate of 24 breaths/min) with shallow breaths. His heart rate was elevated at 92 beats/min, and his blood pressure was low (86/62 mm Hg). His temperature was slightly above normal (38.5℃). Upon auscultation, there were diffuse crackling sounds (rales) in his lung fields. No other abnormalities were observed on physical examination.

Further evaluation revealed a slight reduction in arterial oxygen pressure, evidence of a pleural effusion (fluid around the lungs) on chest radiograph, and indications of right ventricular strain on electrocardiography (ECG). Based on the history of sudden onset of respiratory distress 1 week after major orthopedic surgery and the findings on physical examination, the treating emergency physician suspected a possible pulmonary embolus (PE). To confirm this diagnosis, she ordered a rapid D-dimer blood test, and the result was positive. In addition, a multislice computed tomography study of the chest revealed blockages within multiple pulmonary arteries.

Mr. W. was started immediately on a so-called clot-busting drug, alteplase. The patient also was started on medications to improve cardiac contractions, as well as an anticoagulant. Mr. W. was admitted to the critical care unit, where his symptoms progressively resolved over the next 24 hours. Then he was transferred to a regular nursing care unit, where he was ambulated and was started on a regimen of oral anticoagulant medications and physical therapy along with instruction about preventing recurrence of venous thromboembolism (VTE). He was discharged 3 days later, remaining on oral anticoagulants for 3 months without any further complications.

CLINICAL BACKGROUND

The patient in the Health Scenario had a postoperative PE. A PE is the blockage of one or more pulmonary arteries by a blood clot. Typically, these clots arise in the deep veins of the leg, or less commonly, other parts of the body. Such a clot is referred to as deep vein thrombosis (DVT). Because PEs tend to occur in conjunction with DVTs, the two entities are aggregated together under the rubric VTE.

Trailing only myocardial infarction and stroke, VTE is the third most common life-threatening form of cardiovascular disease in the United States. More than a half million hospitalizations each year in this country are associated with a diagnosis of a VTE.

Because many VTEs occur as an unintended consequence of medical care, groups dedicated to improving patient safety and health care quality have ranked VTE as the most common preventable cause of hospital death in this country.

An understanding of VTE begins with an appreciation of the factors that contribute to the formation of clots (thrombi) in deep veins. Classically, a triad of factors is associated with the genesis of thrombi: (1) diminished venous blood flow, (2) increased coagulability of blood, and (3) damage to the blood vessel wall. A thrombus is a solid accumulation of platelets, fibrin, and trapped red and white blood cells that forms within and blocks a blood vessel. Fragments of the clot, referred to as emboli, may break off and get swept away into the circulation, eventually wedging themselves in the smaller blood vessels of the pulmonary vascular tree. The redistributed blood flow creates areas of low ventilation–perfusion within the lung, resulting in impaired gas exchange.

A number of factors may predispose a patient to experience a VTE. Some of these characteristics are related to an elevation in the risk of clotting. These traits include, among others, advanced age (older than 40 years), a prior history of VTE, cigarette smoking, the use of estrogens or birth control pills, cancer, and certain autoimmune diseases. Other predisposing factors are related to diminished blood flow. These conditions include, but are not limited to, a family history of VTE, obesity, recent surgery (particularly those involving the pelvis, hip, or knee), fracture of the pelvis or legs, bed rest, the postpartum period, and placement of a heart pacemaker through a catheter in the groin.

The symptoms of a DVT may include single-sided leg or thigh redness, warmth, pain, or swelling, but about half of DVTs have no associated symptoms. With PE, the onset of symptoms often is abrupt with shortness of breath and pain when breathing, sometimes associated with a cough or coughing up blood (hemoptysis). Complaints related to DVT may or may not be present. Upon examination, patients with PE often exhibit rapid breathing (tachypnea) accompanied by a rapid heart rate (tachycardia); low blood pressure (hypotension, and if extremely low, shock); fever; and if oxygenation is poor, a pale or bluish skin color.

The history and physical examination can produce a high level of suspicion of a VTE, but the definitive diagnosis requires further studies. For patients in respiratory distress, prompt measurement of arterial oxygenation is essential. A rapid test for D-dimer, a breakdown product of cross-linked fibrin is useful, but it can be elevated in other conditions, as well. An ECG is important to rule out a myocardial infarction but can also provide supporting evidence of right heart dysfunction, as can an echocardiography. Often, chest radiograph results are normal, but they may reveal changes in the pulmonary vascularity, or fluid between the lung and chest wall.

Computed tomography of the chest with injected contrast material may reveal a filling defect in the pulmonary vasculature. Other imaging studies, such as pulmonary angiography and ventilation–perfusion scans, also may be used. DVTs often can be detected by compression ultrasonography, with clots indicated by internal sound echoes and the inability to compress the vein.

An acute, massive PE is a medical emergency, with 3% of patients dying within 48 hours and 10% expiring during hospitalization. The clinical course is particularly ominous for patients who experience shock, respiratory failure, or both. Initial management, therefore, is focused on achieving hemodynamic stability and optimal oxygenation. Medications can be used to increase blood pressure and cardiac output, as necessary. Simultaneously, oxygenation can be enhanced by dissolving the embolus, if it is massive, using clot-busting drugs or by interventional mechanical removal. Further clot formation is prevented by the administration of intravenous anticoagulants followed by maintenance on injectable or oral anticoagulants for a minimum of 3 months. The use of graduated compression stockings and frequent ambulation also helps to reduce the risk of additional clots.

INTRODUCTION

Health care professionals often are confronted with life-threatening situations in which the benefits of a treatment must be weighed against the risks associated with it. In the Health Scenario, for example, the emergency physician must balance the benefits of breaking up the clots in the pulmonary arteries of the patient with the risk of inducing serious bleeding from the use of clot-busting drugs. Although this particular situation involves a relatively extreme comparison of risks and benefits, less dramatic appraisals are made routinely in patient care. In this chapter, we provide an overview of how epidemiologic measures can be used to characterize various outcomes and support evidence-based practice.

MEASURES OF DISEASE OCCURRENCE

Three measures are used to quantify the frequency of events that occur in health care. The first is **risk**, which relates to the likelihood that an event (e.g., disease development or death) will occur. The second is **prevalence**, which corresponds to the proportion of a population that is affected by a disease. Finally, **incidence rate** refers to the speed with which new instances of a disease are developing.

Risk

Risk, sometimes also referred to as cumulative incidence, is an indicator of the proportion of persons within a specified population who develop the outcome of interest (e.g., onset of disease or death), within a defined time period.

We can express this concept in the form of an equation:

$$R = \frac{\text{New cases}}{\text{Persons at risk}} = \frac{A}{N}$$

where R is the estimated risk; A is the number of new instances of the outcome of interest, often described as new cases; and N is the number of unaffected persons at the beginning of the observation period. It is important to emphasize that at the outset, all persons under consideration must be free of the outcome of interest. The risk of developing the outcome then can range anywhere between 0 (if no outcomes occur during the observation period) and 1 (if all unaffected persons become affected during the observation period). For simplicity, risk often is presented as a percentage by multiplying the proportion by 100. The following example illustrates the calculation of risk, and weighing risks and benefits.

Example 1. Vekeman and colleagues (2012) were interested in the risk of VTE after total hip or knee arthroplasty and whether the use of anticoagulants to prevent VTEs might induce an unacceptable number of episodes of serious bleeding. Through a large national database, the investigators were able to identify more than 820,000 inpatient hospital stays for adults age 18 years or older who underwent one of these procedures between 2000 and 2008. A total of 8042 VTEs were observed during these hospital stays. The risk of a VTE among total hip or knee replacement admissions, therefore, is:

$$R = \frac{8042}{820,197} = 0.0098 = 0.98\%$$

In other words, about 1 in 100 patients undergoing these particular orthopedic procedures experienced a VTE during their hospitalizations. Similarly, the risk of a major bleeding event was calculated as:

$$R = \frac{2740}{820,197} = 0.0033 = 0.33\%$$

This means that about 1 in 300 patients undergoing these particular orthopedic procedures experienced a major episode of bleeding during hospitalization. The risk of a clot, therefore, is about three times greater than the risk of a major bleeding episode during the immediate hospitalization. In reaching any definitive conclusion about the full risks and benefits of anticoagulation, however, one would need to consider the period beyond the immediate hospitalization, as well as the outcomes of the thrombotic and bleeding episodes.

Prevalence

*The proportion of persons within a population who have the condition of interest is referred to as **prevalence**.* Sometimes we designate this proportion further as relating to a specific point in time (point prevalence) or alternately, to a particular time period (period prevalence). The prevalence is calculated by dividing the number of affected persons (cases) by the number of persons in the source population. Mathematically, we calculate prevalence as:

$$P = \frac{C}{N}$$

where P is the prevalence, C is the number of cases, and N is the size of the source population. As with risk, prevalence can range from 0 (no persons with the condition of interest), to 1 (everybody in the source population is affected). We can also express prevalence as a percentage, by multiplying by 100. The following example illustrates the calculation of prevalence.

Example 2. Deitelzweig and colleagues (2011) were interested in estimating the prevalence of VTE in the United States. For that purpose, they accessed a database that combined commercial insurance claims with those of Medicare beneficiaries for the 5-year period 2002 to 2006. The source population of these databases included 12.7 million persons. Of these persons, 200,007 had a VTE, so the 5-year period prevalence was:

$$P = \frac{200{,}007}{12.7 \text{ million}} = 0.016 = 1.6\%$$

The investigators calculated the 5-year period prevalence separately for DVT (1.1%), PE (0.4%), and both DVT and PE (0.1%). The annual prevalence of VTE was observed to increase progressively over the 5-year study period, with a low of 0.32% in 2002, rising to a high of 0.42% in 2006. The investigators also demonstrated a strong predilection for VTE among persons aged 65 years and older.

Incidence Rate

The incidence rate measures the rapidity with which newly diagnosed cases of a disease develop. The faster the population is becoming affected, the higher the incidence rate. To estimate the incidence rate, one follows a source population of unaffected persons over time, counting the number of individuals who become newly affected (cases), and expresses it relative to person-time (PT), which is a combination of the size of the source population and the time period of observation.

The quantification of PT may seem a little confusing at first, so let us explore how it is calculated. The goal is to estimate the total amount of disease-free time that subjects in the source population are observed. For example, an individual who is followed for 1 year without developing the condition of interest contributes 1 year of observation. Another person may develop the condition of interest 6 months into the study. Although this individual may be followed for a full year, he or she only contributes a half year of disease-free observation to the study. In this manner, each individual contributes a specific amount of disease-free observation, which then can be summed over all persons in the source population, yielding a total PT of observation. Then, we can calculate the incidence rate as:

$$IR = \frac{A}{PT}$$

where IR is the incidence rate, A is the number of newly diagnosed occurrences of the condition of interest, and PT is the total amount of disease-free observation within the source population.

Example 3. To estimate the incidence rate of VTE in the Canadian province of Québec, Tagalakis and colleagues (2013) accessed health care administrative databases to identify all new cases of DVT or PE between 2000 and 2009. The overall incidence of VTE was found to be:

$$IR = \frac{91{,}761 \text{ cases}}{74{,}297{,}764 \text{ person-year}}$$
$$= 0.001\,24 \text{ cases/person-year}$$

To express the incidence rate with fewer decimal places, it is convenient to convert it to 1.24 cases/1000 person-years of observation. An equivalent expression would be 124 cases per 100,000 person-years of observation. In other words, among residents of the province of Québec during the decade of 2000 to 2009, the overall incidence rate of newly diagnosed VTEs was a little more than one 1000 persons followed for 1 year.

In a large population, such as that of the province of Québec, it would be difficult to enumerate the person-years of observation by summing the amount of observation for each individual person over the entire population. An approximation for the population time can be obtained by multiplying the average size of the population at risk (as estimated through a census) by the length of time the population is observed. The estimate will be reasonably accurate if the condition of interest is relatively infrequent in the general population (as is the case for VTE) and there are no major demographic shifts (e.g., in-migration or out-migration) during the period of observation. It is important to note that the incidence rate relates to the first occurrence of the disease or condition of interest. VTE is a disorder that can recur, so if all episodes of VTE in a population (both initial and recurrent) are counted, the estimate of the VTE incidence rate will be inflated. To avoid this problem, the investigator must be able to exclude prior diagnoses of VTE when identifying incident cases.

DISTINCTIONS BETWEEN MEASURES OF DISEASE FREQUENCY

Risk, prevalence, and incidence rate are among the most commonly used measures in epidemiology and clinical medicine. Unfortunately, they also are often misunderstood and inappropriately used interchangeably. In reality, these terms relate to distinct concepts. As an exercise in understanding the differences between these measures, it may be useful to consider the following illustration.

Example 4. Spencer and colleagues (2009) undertook a population-based study in Worcester, Massachusetts, to determine the incidence rates, clinical features, and outcomes of VTE. The patients were identified from hospital admissions, as well as from outpatient, emergency department, imaging, and

laboratory facilities. First occurrences of VTEs were included for 3 years of diagnoses: 1999, 2001, and 2003. The patients were followed for about 3 years on average for determination of any recurrences.

In all, 1567 incident cases of VTE occurred, which corresponded to an incidence rate of 1.14 cases/1000 person-years, similar but slightly lower than the incidence rate previously noted for Québec province. As shown in **Figure 2-1**, the incidence rate for VTE was strongly age dependent, with the highest rates among elderly adults. Examination of incidence rates by gender (**Figure 2-2**) revealed higher rates among women than among men. Similarly, when incidence rates were examined over time, there was little suggestion of any increase (data not shown).

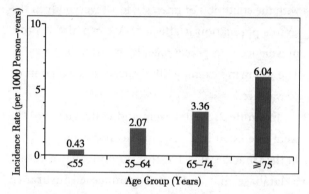

Figure 2-1. Incidence rates of venous thromboembolism, by age, Worcester, Massachusetts, 1999 to 2003. (Data from Emery C, Joffe SW, et al. Incidence rates, clinical profile, and outcomes of patients with venous thromboembolism. The Worcester VTE Study. J Thromb Thrombolysis. 2009;28:401-409.)

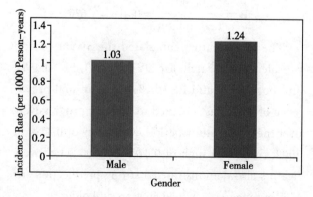

Figure 2-2. Incidence rates of venous thromboembolism, by gender, Worcester, Massachusetts, 1999 to 2003. (Data from Spencer FA, Emery C, Joffe SW, et al. Incidence rates, clinical profile, and outcomes of patients with venous thromboembolism. The Worcester VTE Study. J Thromb Thrombolysis. 2009;28:401-409.)

When the medical characteristics of these patients at the time of VTE diagnosis were considered, the prevalence of a recent (within 3 months) surgery was:

$$P = \frac{478 \text{ recent surgeries}}{1567 \text{ VTE patients}} = 0.305 = 30.5\%$$

Similarly, the prevalence of a recent (within 3 months) central venous catheterization was:

$$P = \frac{312 \text{ recent catheterizations}}{1567 \text{ VTE patiens}} = 0.199 = 19.9\%$$

The risk of developing a recurrent VTE within an average follow-up period of about 3 years was:

$$R = \frac{260 \text{ recurrences}}{1567 \text{ VTE patients}} = 0.166 = 16.6\%$$

Over the same follow-up period, the risk of developing major bleeding on anticoagulant therapy was:

$$R = \frac{194 \text{ bleeding episodes}}{1567 \text{ VTE patients}} = 0.124 = 12.4\%$$

In this single study, the investigators have characterized aspects of VTE occurrence using all three types of measures of disease frequency. They used incidence rates to characterize the rapidity with which VTE was arising within the population of Worcester, Massachusetts. They further characterized patterns of occurrence by examining incidence rates by age, gender, and time period. They then described the clinical profile of the VTE-affected individuals at diagnosis by examining the prevalence of various risk factors of disease occurrence, such as recent surgery or central catheterization. Finally, they estimated the risk of subsequent adverse events, such as recurrent VTEs or bleeding, by following the patients over time to determine the percentage who experienced these complications. Each of these measures helps to complete the picture of the pattern of occurrence of VTE within the population.

SURVIVAL

For diseases, such as VTE, that can have serious impacts on an affected person's well-being, we may wish to characterize the likelihood of remaining alive, or survival, after a diagnosis. Mathematically, we would measure survival (S) as:

$$S = \frac{A-D}{A}$$

where A is the number of newly diagnosed patients with the condition of interest and D is the number of deaths. Survival is, therefore, a proportion that can range from 0 (when no patients survive) to 1 (when all patients survive). We can convert survival to a percentage by multiplying by 100. It is important to recognize that survival is a time-dependent phenomenon, therefore, it is essential to specify a time period for the measurement of survival, such as the 30-day survival, or the 1-year survival.

Example 5. In the previously cited study by Tagalakis and colleagues (2013) of VTE in Québec province, patients were followed for survival after their initial diagnosis. Among the 33,447 persons with a PE, there were 5654 deaths within the first 30 days after diagnosis. The 30-day survival, therefore, is calculated as:

$$S = \frac{33,447 - 5654}{33,447} = 0.83 = 83\%$$

Survival estimates provide a clear and meaningful way to characterize the prognosis of a condition. For example, in this same study population, among the 58,314 persons with a newly diagnosed DVT, the 30-day survival estimate was 93%. As shown in **Figure 2-3**, the near-term (30 day) prognosis after PE is worse (lower survival) than that for DVT. For both PE and DVT, the likelihood of surviving the first 30 days was highly related to the patient's age at diagnosis. The age-specific survival estimates are shown for PE in **Figure 2-4**. It can be seen from this graph that persons age 80 years or older have almost a one third lower probability of surviving for 1 month after a PE than persons 40 years or younger. Thus, some basic information about the diagnosis and the personal characteristics of the patient can be helpful in predicting the clinical outcome.

It should be emphasized that although these likelihoods are derived from the experiences of a group of patients, they also represent our best predictions for an individual patient who fits within the corresponding group. In other words, the evidence from this investigation suggests that among a group of persons 80 years or older with a new PE, 71% will survive for at least 1 month after diagnosis. Similarly, our best estimate from these data of the 30-day survival rate for an individual 82-year-old patient with a new PE is 71%.

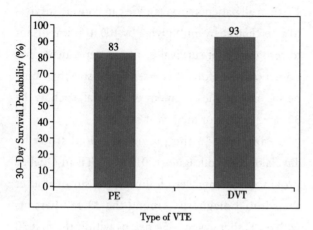

Figure 2-3. Thirty-day survival after a venous thromboembolism (VTE), by type (pulmonary embolus [PE] or deep vein thrombosis [DVT]), Québec province, 2000 to 2009. (Data from Tagalakis V, Patenaude V, Kahn SR, Suissa S. Incidence of and mortality from venous thromboembolism in a real-world population: the Q-VTE Study Cohort. Am J Med. 2013;126:832.e13-21.)

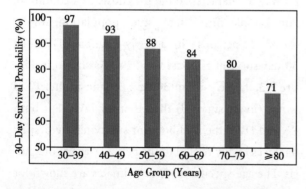

Figure 2-4. Thirty-day survival probabilities after a diagnosis of pulmonary embolus, by age at onset. (Data from Tagalakis V, Patenaude V, Kahn SR, Suissa S. Incidence of and mortality from venous thromboembolism in a real-world population: the Q-VTE Study Cohort. Am J Med. 2013;126:832.e13-21.)

When the survival period of interest is relatively short, such as 30 days, the likelihood that one will be able to follow all patients to the end of the observation period is quite high. On the other hand, as the duration of the follow-up period increases, so does the likelihood that the investigator will not be able to

track each and every subject for the full time period. For example, a patient may move away from the study area. In studies in which individual patients are being tracked for their outcomes, subjects may be lost to observation for a variety of reasons, such as relocation, changing names (through marriage or other circumstances), voluntarily withdrawing from participation, or because the study ends before the patient has completed the full observation period of interest. If such losses are substantial, excluding these patients with incomplete follow-up might introduce error in estimation, which we refer to as a bias. Consider for instance, that patients who move away have more favorable outcomes than those who remain. Excluding those subjects who relocate, therefore, would yield an erroneously low estimate of survival. Even if the outcomes do not differ, throwing out all information on patients who were lost to follow-up is wasteful in a statistical sense. By this, we mean that reducing the number of subjects under consideration is tantamount to reducing the sample size, and as a consequence, our survival estimates are not as precise as they might otherwise be if these individuals were included.

Fortunately, there are statistical techniques that allow an investigator to use all of the follow-up information that is available, even for patients who are lost to follow-up or for whom the study ends before they complete the full follow-up period. Two such techniques are life-table analysis and so-called Kaplan-Meier analysis. Although the methods for performing these calculations are beyond the scope of this discussion, readers who are interested in more detail may consult discussions of survival analysis in most biostatistics textbooks.

Survival results over time often are depicted in a graphical format, such as that shown in **Figure 2-5.** Here survival likelihood is shown for the first 2 years after a new VTE diagnosis among persons who also had cancer. On the horizontal axis, time since the first diagnosis of the VTE is depicted in months, with 0 time representing when the diagnosis was made. Over time, the percentage of persons surviving declines, with key observation periods every

6 months. It can be seen that the most dramatic decrease in survival occurs in the first 6 months after a VTE, with smaller risk of death in subsequent observation periods.

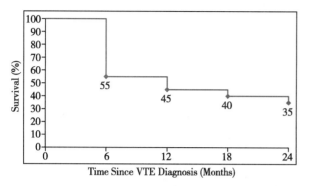

Figure 2-5. Survival curve from the time of an incident venous thromboembolism (VTE) diagnosis for persons with preexisting cancer.

Example 6. One might want to summarize the survival results with a single measure, such as the percentage of persons with cancer surviving for 2 years after a first VTE. To estimate this probability as shown in **Figure 2-6**, one first goes to the follow-up period of interest—in this case, 24 months—and draws a vertical line (A) to the survival curve. From the point at which line A intersects the survival curve, one draws a horizontal line (B) to the y axis. The point of intersection of line B with the y axis yields the survival probability—in this case, 35%.

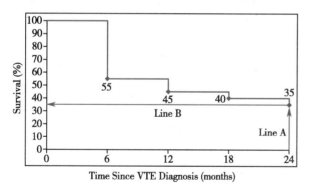

Figure 2-6. Approach to estimating the 2-year survival probability after a venous thromboembolism (VTE) diagnosis among persons with cancer.

Another useful measure to characterize the observed survival experience is the **median survival time**. This corresponds to the amount of time after diagnosis at which point half of the affected individuals remain alive. **Figure 2-7** shows how the median survival time is estimated. First, one draws a horizontal line from 50% survival on the y axis to the survival curve. From the point at which line A intersects the survival curve, one draws a vertical line (B) to the x axis. The point of intersection of line B with the x axis yields the median survival time—in this case, 12 months.

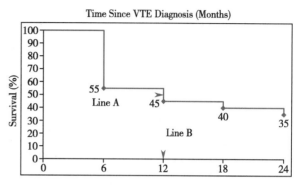

Figure 2-7. Approach to estimating the median survival time after a venous thromboembolism (VTE) diagnosis among persons with cancer.

Case-Fatality

Another measure of prognosis after a diagnosis is the **case fatality**. *This metric refers to the proportion (or percentage) of persons with a particular condition who die within a specified period of time.* Often, case-fatality is incorrectly referred to as a rate or a ratio, but it is more accurately described as a risk or probability. It is calculated mathematically as:

$$CF = \frac{\text{Number of deaths}}{\text{Number of diagnosed persons}} = \frac{D}{A}$$

where CF is case-fatality, D is the number of deaths, and A is the number of persons with the condition of interest. The case-fatality can range from 0 when there are no deaths observed during the specified timeframe to 1 when all affected persons with the condition of interest die during the specified timeframe. For simplicity, the case-fatality often is expressed as a percentage by multiplying by 100.

Example 7. The previously cited study of VTE in Québec province (Tagalakis et al, 2013) included information on case-fatality risks at 30 days and 1 year after diagnosis. The results are shown separately for DVTs and PEs in **Figure 2-8**. It can be seen that PEs have a much higher associated risk of death than do DVTs, with the excess appearing soon after the diagnosis and persisting through subsequent observation.

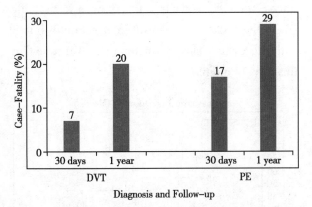

Figure 2-8. Case-fatality percentages at 30 days and 1 year after diagnosis for deep vein thrombosis (DVT) and pulmonary embolus (PE), Québec province, 2000 to 2009. (Data from Tagalakis V, Patenaude V, Kahn SR, Suissa S. Incidence of and mortality from venous thromboembolism in a real-world population: the Q-VTE Study Cohort. Am J Med. 2013;126:832.e13-21.)

Because case-fatality reflects the probability of death within a defined period of time and survival relates to the probability of not dying in that defined period, the two measures may be thought of as inverse proportions—as one increases, the other, of necessity, decreases.

Mortality rate

Mortality rate is a measure of the number of deaths (in general, or due to a specific cause) in a particular population, scaled to the size of that population, per unit of time. The computation of mortality rate is based on similar equations as incidence rate. The numerator therefore contains the number of death instead of the number of cases:

$$MR = \frac{D}{PT}$$

where MR is the mortality rate, D is the number of deaths, and PT is the total amount of observation (whether diagnosed or not) within the source population.

Example 8. The previously cited Worcester VTE study (Spencer et al, 2013) provided case-fatality rate of the 1999 cohort (CF = 43.3%), so we can figure out the number of deaths (D) during the 1216 days '

follow-up time(3.33 years) as:

D = Number of diagnosed persons × CF = 499
 × 43.3% = 216

Then we calculate the mortality rate of VTE as follows:

$$MR = \frac{216 \text{ deaths}}{477,800 \times 3.33 \text{ person-year}}$$
$$= 13.6 \text{ cases}/100,000 \text{ person-years}$$

In other words, among the greater Worcester population during the observation time, more than 13 persons out of 100 thousand died from VTE.

SUMMARY

In this chapter, we featured basic measures of disease frequency and prognosis. Each of these metrics is used commonly in epidemiology and clinical medicine. Despite their routine appearance in the literature, the meaning and appropriate application of these measures often is misconstrued. To review, **risk** (also referred to as cumulative incidence) is the fraction of unaffected individuals within a defined population who newly develop the condition of interest during a specified time period. **Prevalence** also is defined as a proportion, but it refers to the fraction of persons within a population who have the condition of interest at any particular point or period of time. **Incidence rate** refers to the rapidity with which unaffected persons within a defined population develop the condition of interest. Risk, prevalence, and incidence rate are used typically to quantify the amount, sometimes called burden, of disease within a particular group of people. Several measures are used to characterize the prognosis of a condition of interest after it has occurred. Risk can be used to characterize the likelihood that a particular outcome (favorable or unfavorable) will occur among newly affected persons with the condition of interest over a specified period of time. **Survival** is the probability of a particular outcome (remaining alive) during a specified period of time after diagnosis with the condition of interest. **Case-fatality** is the inverse of survival and represents the likelihood of a particular outcome (death) during a specified time period after diagnosis of the condition of interest. **Mortality rate** is another measure of disease burden, which represents the amount of deaths in a given general population during a given period of time.

We have seen how each of these measures can be used to help quantify aspects of VTE occurrence and prognosis. Specifically, we learned that whereas the risk of a VTE arising during the hospitalization for a total knee or hip replacement was about 1%, the risk of a major bleeding episode on routine anticoagulant therapy to prevent VTEs was one third as great. The 5-year period prevalence of VTE in the United States was shown to be between 1% and 2% of the general population. The incidence rate of VTE separately was found to be slightly more than one case for every 1000 person-years of observation. We learned that the incidence rate of VTE is highly related to age, with the highest rates among elderly adults. Among patients with a newly diagnosed VTE, the prevalence of recent surgery was almost one third, and the prevalence of a recent central venous catheterization was about one fifth.

In terms of prognosis, we learned that the risk of recurrence of a VTE over 3 years was about one in six patients, and the risk of a major bleeding episode was about one in eight patients. We also learned that whereas a particularly serious form of VTE, PE, has a 30-day survival probability of only 83%, those diagnosed with a DVT had a 1-month survival probability of 93%. We also saw that survival probability was strongly related to age, with 30-day survival from PE much more likely among young adults. What's more, we found that the case-fatality percentage at 1 year after diagnosis of a PE was much higher (29%) than the corresponding 1-year case-fatality for DVT (20%). Finally, we speculate that the mortality rate of VTE was 13.6/100,000 person-years.

Together, these measures have painted a very clear picture of VTE in the general population. This is a common condition, with particularly high risk among persons undergoing invasive medical procedures. The prognosis is strongly related to the type of VTE and the age of the patient at diagnosis, with sig-nificant loss of life in the first month after diagnosis.

(Xiaoping Miao)

IMPORTANT TERMINOLOGY

risk	风险
prevalence	患病率
point prevalence	时点患病率
period prevalence	期间患病率
incidence rate	发病率
survival	生存率
survival analysis	生存分析
life-table	寿命表
median survival time	中位生存期
case-fatality	病死率
mortality rate	死亡率
bias	偏倚

 STUDY QUESTIONS

1. *To characterize the burden of diabetes mellitus on a population, an investigator conducts a household survey of residents. The most appropriate measure in this context is*

   A. *risk.*

   B. *prevalence.*

   C. *incidence rate.*

   D. *survival.*

   E. *case-fatality.*

   F. *mortality rate.*

2. *To assess prognosis after a diagnosis of diabetic coma, an investigator collects information on deaths within 30 days. The most appropriate measure in this context is*

   A. *cumulative incidence.*

   B. *prevalence.*

   C. *incidence rate.*

   D. *attributable risk.*

   E. *case-fatality.*

   F. *mortality rate.*

3. *To assess the likelihood of women developing diabetes during pregnancy, an investigator follows 10,000 nondiabetic women from inception to completion of pregnancy and determines the percent-age of them who develop gestational diabetes. The most appropri-*

ate measure in this context is

A. cumulative incidence.

B. prevalence.

C. incidence rate.

D. attributable risk.

E. case-fatality.

F. mortality rate.

4. *To assess the rapidity with which diabetes mellitus develops among a cohort of morbidly obese young adults, an investigator follows each non-diabetic obese student for the development of newly diagnosed diabetes mellitus from matriculation at a university through graduation. The most appropriate measure in this context is*

A. cumulative incidence.

B. prevalence.

C. incidence rate.

D. attributable risk.

E. case-fatality.

F. mortality rate.

5. *Which of the following measures may be thought of as the inverse of case-fatality?*

A. Cumulative incidence

B. Prevalence

C. Incidence rate

D. Survival

E. Attributable risk

F. Mortality rate

FURTHER READING

Heit JA. The epidemiology of venous thromboembolism in the community. *Arterioscler Thromb Vasc Biol.* 2008;28:370-372.

Wong P, Baglin T. Epidemiology, risk factors and sequelae of venous thromboembolism. *Phlebology.* 2012;27(suppl 2): 2-11.

REFERENCES

Clinical Background

Pollak AW, McBane RD. Succinct review of the new VTE

prevention and management guidelines. *Mayo Clin Proc.* 2014;89:394-408.

Wells PS, Forgie MA, Rodger MA. Treatment of venous thrombo-embolism. *JAMA.* 2014;311:717-728.

Risk

Vekeman F, LaMori JC, Laliberté F, et al. In-hospital risk of venous thromboembolism and bleeding and associated costs for patients undergoing total hip or knee arthroplasty. *J Med Econ.* 2012;15:644-653.

Prevalence

Deitelzweig SB, Johnson BH, Lin J, Schulman KL. Prevalence of clinical venous thromboembolism in the USA: current trends and future projections. *Am J Hematol.* 2011;86:217-220.

Incidence

Tagalakis V, Patenaude V, Kahn SR, Suissa S. Incidence of and mortality from venous thromboembolism in a real-world population: the Q-VTE Study Cohort. *Am J Med.* 2013;126(832):e13-21.

Distinctions Between Measures of Disease Frequency

Spencer FA, Emery C, Joffe SW, et al. Incidence rates, clinical profile, and outcomes of patients with venous thromboembolism. The Worcester VTE Study. *J Thromb Thrombolysis.* 2009; 28:401-409.

Survival

Tagalakis V, Patenaude V, Kahn SR, Suissa S. Incidence of and mortality from venous thromboembolism in a real-world population: the Q-VTE Study Cohort. *Am J Med.* 2013;126(832):e13-21.

Case-Fatality

Tagalakis V, Patenaude V, Kahn SR, Suissa S. Incidence of and mortality from venous thromboembolism in a real-world population: the Q-VTE Study Cohort. *Am J Med.* 2013;126(832):e13-21.

Mortality rate

Spencer FA, Emery C, Joffe SW, et al. Incidence rates, clinical profile, and outcomes of patients with venous thromboembolism. The Worcester VTE Study. *J Thromb Thrombolysis.* 2009; 28:401-409.

Global Burden of Disease

HEALTH SCENARIO

At 4:53 pm on Tuesday, January 12, 2010, an earthquake measuring 7.0 on the Richter scale hit Haiti. The earthquake was the most powerful to strike the island in more than 200 years, and it was centered near the capital city, Port-au-Prince, where a quarter of the nation's nearly 10 million citizens lived.

The devastation caused by the earthquake was severe, with an estimated 250,000 residences and 30,000 commercial buildings either collapsed or severely damaged. The exact number of fatalities was uncertain, but the death toll was estimated to be 200,000 to 300,000, with another 300,000 non-fatal injuries. The number of displaced persons was estimated to be 1.3 million, with nearly 400,000 still residing in temporary shelters a year and a half after the earthquake.

The catastrophic dimensions of the earthquake can be attributed to a number of factors. Haiti is a very poor country, with 80% of its citizens living under the poverty level. As a consequence of the economic conditions, buildings there are poorly designed, constructed, and inspected. Construction materials are of inferior quality, and many buildings are sited on hillsides without adequate structural support. Moreover, the earthquake was centered in a densely populated area, increasing the number of people affected.

The tragedy of the earthquake was compounded by the logistical challenges of getting relief workers and supplies into the country. In addition, nearly two thirds of Haiti's hospitals were destroyed by the earthquake, adversely impacting the speed and capacity of the medical response.

The devastation caused by the earthquake was followed 10 months later by an outbreak of cholera. This epidemic began in a region about 100 km north of Port-au-Prince, with the source presumed to be drinking water drawn from a contaminated river. Because three out of four Haitian households lack running water and sanitation conditions are poor, the disease was easily transmitted from person to person. Within 10 weeks, the disease had spread throughout the country, ultimately affecting 6% of all Haitians. Hundreds of thousands of persons were hospitalized, and more than 3000 deaths were reported within 2 months. New cases were still arising years after the outbreak, with peaks occurring during the rainy season and after hurricanes.

The earthquake and ensuing cholera epidemic in Haiti demonstrate dramatically that death and disability from natural disasters and communicable diseases still burden substantial human populations, particularly those in economically challenged parts of the world. In this chapter, we will examine general patterns of health and disease throughout the world, with a focus on variations across person, place, and time.

GLOBAL BURDEN OF DISEASE STUDY

Imagine an effort to characterize the distribution and determinants of human health and disease around the world. Such an undertaking would require a large number of data sources; a highly collaborative, interdisciplinary team of investigators; extensive computational resources; complicated protocols and analyses; and substantial financial investment. All of these elements were brought together in a monumental effort referred to as the Global **Burden of Disease** Study 2010 (GBD 2010). The purpose of the GBD 2010 was to measure the relative amounts of health loss resulting from diseases, injuries, and **risk factors**, with **assessment** of trends over time, place, and personal attributes. After being assembled, this information can be applied for the following purposes:

1. To better understand the leading contributors to losses in human health and to describe how these contributions vary by person, place, and time

2. To help set priorities for initiatives to promote human health

3. To measure progress in addressing the leading health problems worldwide

4. To identify gaps in information on human health in order to improve the quality and quantity of data available

The GBD 2010, by virtue of its size, scale, rigor, and complexity, has set a new standard for descriptive epidemiology at the international level.

Study Design

The GBD 2010 followed three earlier versions in 1990, 1999 to 2002, and 2004. GBD 2010 greatly expanded the prior studies by including more diseases, more risk factors, more age groups, and multiple time periods. GBD 2010 was undertaken as a partnership between seven primary institutions: the University of Washington, Harvard University, Johns Hopkins University, the University of Queensland, Imperial College of London, the University of Tokyo, and the World Health Organization. The collaborative team of investigators included 486 scientists from 302 institutions in 50 counties.

The study was initiated in 2007 and was completed 5 years later. About 100,000 sources of data were identified by a systematic search for potential use in deriving estimates of the burden of disease. The resulting database contained information on 800 million deaths between 1950 and 2010. A major challenge in assembling the database was the fact that

vital registration systems that include medical certification are not established in many countries, particularly those in the developing world. For example, in a recent year, only 36% of all deaths occurred in countries using physician certification. Even when medical input is required, comparisons across countries may be affected by varying skills of physicians, variability in information available at the time the death certificate is completed, differing practices in assigning underlying causes of death, and other legal and procedural issues.

For deaths that are not medically certified, a variety of other sources of information were used, including, among others, surveillance systems, disease registries, demographic surveys, and police reports. The diversity of data origins and potential errors associated with them contribute to uncertainty in the resulting death rates. Ranges of uncertainty were presented for estimated measures in the results. Because the emphasis of the present summary is to capture the major patterns and trends, only the best estimates are reported here. GBD 2010 used a list of 291 diseases and injuries and 1160 sequelae of these conditions, the latter being defined as the direct consequences of disease or injury that were not otherwise captured. In addition, 67 risk factors for disease were estimated. Separate estimates of outcomes were made for 187 individual countries. These countries were also grouped into 21 regions based on demographic similarity and geographic proximity, and outcomes were estimated for these regions.

The computational requirements for GBD 2010 were enormous. Using a network of more than 100 computers, the amount of data stored after a modeling process could exceed 3 terabytes of information. The human effort of summarizing and interpreting these results was similarly demanding.

Mortality

There were 52.8 million deaths in the world in 2010. This represents an increase of 6.3 million deaths (13.5%) compared with the number of death in 1990. The rise in the number of deaths does not imply that human health declined during this 20-year period. In reality, age-standardized death rates declined by 21.5% during this interval.

The seemingly paradoxical rise in the number of deaths occurred because the population grew and aged between 1990 and 2010. As shown in Figure 3-1, if the population size and age composition had remained unchanged and the 1990 death rates had continued in 2010, an extra 8.5 million deaths would have occurred. A further 9 million deaths would have occurred in 2010 if the 1990 death rates applied to the larger and older world population in 2010.

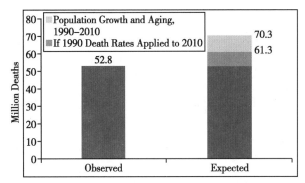

Figure 3-1. Observed numbers of deaths in the world, 2010. Expected numbers were calculated using the 1990 death rates and separately accounting for the aging and growth of the population between 1990 and 2010. (Data from Lozano R, Pourmalek F, Raju M, et al. Global and regional mortality from 235 causes of death for 20 age groups in 1990 and 2010: a systematic analysis for the Global Burden of Disease Study 2010. Lancet. 2012;380:2095-2128.)

The 10 leading causes of death in 2010 are shown in Table 3-1 along with the respective age-standardized mortality rates. Collectively, these leading causes of death account for more than half of all deaths and more than half of the overall age-standardized mortality rate. Six of the top 10 causes of death, including the top three, are noncommunicable diseases or injuries. Compared with the corresponding ranking 2 decades earlier, the most dramatic increases were the rise of HIV/AIDS (rank 35 to 6), diabetes (rank 15 to 9), lung cancer (rank 8 to 5), and road injuries (rank 10 to 8). The largest declines in ranking during this 20-year interval were seen for preterm birth complications (rank 7 to 15), tuberculosis (rank 6 to 10), diarrhea (rank 5 to 7), and lower respiratory infections (rank 3 to 4).

Table 3-1 The 10 leading causes of death in 2010 along with the age-standardized mortality rates

Cause	Age-Standardized Mortality Rate[a]
1. Ischemic heart disease	105.7
2. Stroke	88.4
3. Chronic obstructive pulmonary disease	43.8
4. Lower respiratory infections	41.0
5. Lung cancer	23.4
6. HIV/AIDS	21.4
7. Diarrheal disease	20.9
8. Road injuries	19.5
9. Diabetes	19.5
10. Tuberculosis	18.0

[a]Per 100,000 persons.

Data from Lozano R, et al. Lozano R, Pourmalek F, Raju M, et al. Global and regional mortality from 235 causes of death for 20 age groups in 1990 and 2010: a systematic analysis for the Global Burden of Disease Study 2010. *Lancet.* 2012;380:2095-2128.

To the extent that declining age-standardized mortality rates reflect progress in controlling diseases, some of the more dramatic success stories are shown in Figure 3-2. It is noteworthy that four of the top five cause-specific declines in mortality are related to the control of infectious diseases. These changes reflect the so-called epidemiologic transition in which improvements in nutrition, sanitation, immunization, and medical care in developing nations led to a reduction in mortality from infectious diseases, with consequent growth and aging of the population and a rise in degenerative and human-made diseases.

The list of causes of death with increasing age-adjusted death rates between 1990 and 2010 is far more limited (data not shown). By far, the most dramatic rise in mortality was for HIV/AIDS, with the death rate climbing nearly 260% during this 2-decade period. More modest elevations also were seen for neurologic disorders (38%) and diabetes (20%).

The epidemiologic transition is associated with declines in childhood deaths principally because of the fall of fatal infectious diseases, with a concomitant rise in deaths among adults, attributable primarily to increases in degenerative and human-made diseases. This pattern was observed in GBD 2010, as shown in Figure 3-3.

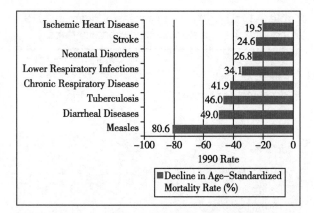

Figure 3-2. Percent declines in age-standardized mortality rates, 1990 to 2010, for selected causes of death. (Data from Lozano R, Pourmalek F, Raju M, et al. Global and regional mortality from 235 causes of death for 20 age groups in 1990 and 2010: a systematic analysis for the Global Burden of Disease Study 2010. Lancet. 2012;380:2095-2128.)

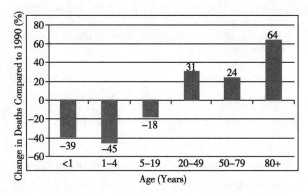

Figure 3-3. Percent change in numbers of deaths by age group, 2010 versus 1990. (Data Lindgren L, Lofgren KT, et al. Age-specific and sex-specific mortality in 187 countries, 1970-analysis for the Global Burden of Disease Study 2010. Lancet. 2012;380:2071-2094.)

Life Expectancy

Estimated age-specific death rates were used to estimate likelihoods of surviving each age period, and ultimately the number of years a person is expected to live from a particular baseline age. For simplicity, life expectancy at birth was used as a summary measure. In 2010, the life expectancy at birth was 67.5 years for males and 73.3 years for females. During the 20-year interval between 1990 and 2010, the life expectancy at birth increased 4.7 years for males and 5.2 years for females.

In 2010, there was considerable variation in life expectancy across different regions of the world. Among females, the region with the greatest life expectancy at birth (High Income Pacific) had an almost 27-year advantage over the region with the lowest life expectancy at birth (Central sub-Saharan Africa). For males, the range of life expectancies between the highest region (Australasia) and the lowest region (central sub-Saharan Africa) was more than 25 years. Table 3-2 shows the four countries with the highest and the four countries with the lowest life expectancies at birth in 2010 by sex. The countries with the longest lived populations are the same for males and females, although the rankings differ slightly. All of these countries are located in the high-income regions of Asia and Western Europe.

The counties with the shortest life expectancies at birth and their rank order are the same for males and females (Table 3-2). These countries are located in the low-income regions of the Caribbean and sub-Saharan Africa. The low life expectancies in sub-Saharan African countries reflect the severe impact of HIV/AIDS in these populations. The low life expectancy in Haiti is attributable to the earthquake that ravaged the country in 2010.

Table 3-2 The four countries with the highest and lowest life expectancies at birth, 2010, by sex

Males		Females	
Highest Life Expectancies			
Iceland	80.0	Japan	85.9
Andorra	79.8	Andorra	85.2
Switzerland	79.7	Switzerland	84.5
Japan	79.3	Iceland	84.4
Lowest Life Expectancies			
Swaziland	47.4	Swaziland	51.4
Lesotho	44.1	Lesotho	50.7
Central African		Central African	
Republic	43.6	Republic	49.3
Haiti	32.5	Haiti	43.6

Data from Wang H, Dwyer-Lindgren L, Lofgren KT, et al. Age-specific and sex-specific mortality in 187 countries, 1970-2010: a systematic analysis for the Global Burden of Disease Study 2010. *Lancet.* 2012;380:2071-2094.

Healthy Life Expectancy

As noted already, progress has been made in virtually all countries toward reducing death rates, with concomitant increases in life expectancy for both males and females. The aging of the population is accompanied by a rise in degenerative and human-made diseases, many of which have considerable morbidities. A reasonable question, therefore, is what proportion of the additional years of life are characterized by good health (i.e., a lack of disability and functional limitations)? In GBD 2010, an attempt was made to address this question by calculation of healthy life expectancy. This measure corresponds to the number of years a person can be anticipated to live in good health beyond some baseline age. To calculate healthy life expectancy, one needs to account for age-specific death rates, **morbidity**, and limitations in functional status.

A particularly challenging aspect of this analysis was to calculate the years lived with disability. To make the best possible determinations, the investigators calculated the prevalence of 1160 sequelae of disease by age, sex, country, and year. More than 100,000 data sources were used to help derive these estimates. The GBD 2010 study had many strengths, such as the use of a wide range of data, and when possible, the incorporation of biomarkers and functional measurement as well as the assessment of severity of impairment. Nevertheless, it must be appreciated that there is considerable uncertainty involved in the estimates of years lived with disability.

Figure 3-4 depicts the total and healthy life expectancies at birth in 2010 for the world by sex. For males, the life expectancy of 67.5 years includes 59.0 years (87.4%) of healthy life. For females, the expected life span of 73.3 years includes 63.2 years (86.2%) of healthy life. Between 1990 and 2010, 4.2 of the 4.7 years gained in life expectancy for males were healthy years. Of the 5.2 years of additional life for females, 4.5 were healthy years.

As with life expectancy, considerable variation existed in the distribution of healthy life expectan-cies (Table 3-3). The highest levels were seen in Japan for both males and females, with the leading nations coming from the high-income Pacific and Western European regions. Haiti again had the lowest levels for both males and females, with the same three sub-Saharan African nations that trailed in life expectancy at birth also having low levels of healthy life. The most extreme contrast of experience between the highest and lowest ranking nations revealed about a 4-decade longer healthy life expectancy at birth for natives of Japan compared with Haitians.

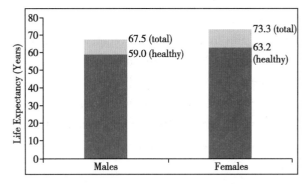

Figure 3-4. Life expectancy at birth and healthy life expectancy at birth (dark shaded) in the world, 2010. (Data from Salomon JA, Wang H, Freeman MK, et al. Healthy life expectancy for 187 countries, 1990-2010: a systematic analysis for the Global Burden of Disease Study 2010. Lancet. 2012;380:2144-2162.)

Table 3-3 The four countries with the highest and lowest healthy life expectancies at birth, 2010, by sex

Males		Females	
Highest Healthy Life Expectancies			
Japan	70.6	Japan	75.5
Singapore	69.6	Spain	73.0
Switzerland	69.1	South Korea	72.6
Spain	68.8	Singapore	72.6
Lowest Healthy Life Expectancies			
Swaziland	40.4	Swaziland	43.3
Lesotho	37.7	Lesotho	42.6
Central African		Central African	
Republic	37.7	Republic	41.7
Haiti	27.8	Haiti	37.1

Data from Salomon JA, Wang H, Freeman MK, et al. Healthy life expectancy for 187 countries, 1990-2010: a systematic analysis for the Global Burden of Disease Study 2010. *Lancet.* 2012;380:2144-2162.

In all but two of the 21 regions of the world, healthy life expectancy at birth increased between 1990 and 2010. The two regions that experienced declines were the Caribbean because of the 2010 earthquake in Haiti and Southern sub-Saharan Africa because of HIV/AIDS. Most of the loss of healthy life expectancy of about 6 years in both of these two regions was attributable to increased deaths in persons age 5 years or older. In Eastern Europe, a small decrease in deaths among children younger than 5 years of age was offset by an increase in mortality among older persons, resulting in minimal change in healthy life expectancy. For the remaining 18 regions, gains in healthy life expectancy ranged from 2 to more than 6 years, with improvements driven by reductions in mortality in the first 5 years of life, among older persons, or a combination of both. There was little contribution to improved healthy life expectancy as a result of diminished disability in any of these regions.

Disability-Adjusted Life Years

Healthy life expectancy provides a convenient summary measure of a population's health status. Disability-adjusted life years (DALYs) provide another way of characterizing the burden of disease within a population. The concept of DALYs was developed initially by the investigators of the first GBD Study in 1990. In brief, DALYs combine information on two components: years of life lost because of premature death and years lived with disability. The years of life lost are determined against the most favorable life expectancy, which is derived by applying the lowest observed age-specific death rates in the world. By summing together lost years of life and years lived with disability, DALYs provide a summary measure of the absolute loss of health due to death or nonfatal illness and are influenced, therefore, by the size and demographic features of the population.

In 2010, there were 2.49 billion DALYs in the world. Premature mortality accounted for more than two thirds (69%) of the loss of healthy life, with the reminder (31%) related to disabilities. The proportion of DALYs related to disabilities has increased over time, reflecting a gradual shift in the burden of disease from rapidly fatal causes to more chronic conditions. As depicted in Figure 3-5, more than half of all DALYs were attributable to noncommunicable diseases; another third coming from communicable, maternal, infant, and nutritional diseases; and the remainder attributable to injuries.

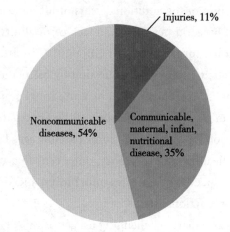

Figure 3-5. Distribution of disability-adjusted life years according to broad groupings of causes, 2010. (Data from Murray CJL, Vos T, Lozano R, et al. Disabilityadjusted life years (DALYs) for 291 diseases and injuries in 21 regions, 1990-2010: a systematic analysis for the Global Burden of Disease Study 2010. Lancet. 2012;380:2197-2223.)

Some of the leading noncommunicable diseases contributing to DALYs are shown in Figure 3-6. The top three diseases—cancer, heart disease, and stroke—were all major causes of death and therefore were responsible for premature loss of life. This contrasts with two of the other leading noncommunicable disease contributors to DALYs—low back pain and depression—which impacted the population primarily as sources of disability.

The DALYs for the five leading communicable diseases are shown in Figure 3-7. These same five diseases were the top causes of death, but the relative lethality varies: HIV/AIDS is ranked second as a cause of death given that it is more likely to be fatal than either malaria or diarrheal disease. Beyond the infectious diseases and the chronic degenerative conditions, other leading contributors to DALYs include preterm birth complications (77.0 million DALYs) and road injuries (75.5 million DALYs).

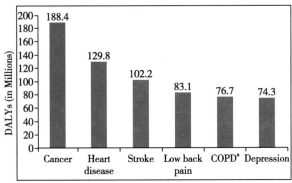

Figure 3-6. Disability-adjusted life years (DALYs) related to leading noncommunicable diseases, 2010. (Data from Murray CJL, Vos T, Lozano R, et al. Disability-adjusted life years (DALYs) for 291 diseases and injuries in 21 regions, 1990-2010: a systematic analysis for the Global Burden of Disease Study 2010. Lancet. 2012;380:2197-2223.)

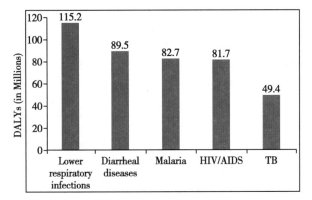

Figure 3-7. Disability-adjusted life years (DALYs) related to leading communicable diseases, 2010. TB, tuberculosis. (Data from Murray CJL, Vos T, Lozano R, et al. Disability-adjusted life years (DALYs) for 291 diseases and injuries in 21 regions, 1990-2010: a systematic analysis for the Global Burden of Disease Study 2010. Lancet. 2012;380:2197-2223.)

Over time, the burden of disease has shifted from the youngest age groups to older persons. For example, in 1990, children younger than 5 years of age accounted for 41% of DALYs. By 2010, the corresponding percentage had dropped to 25%. This dramatic decline in DALYs among children was driven by reductions over time in the two leading causes of DALYs in 1990, lower respiratory infections (44% fall by 2010) and diarrheal diseases (51%). Because four fifths of these illnesses occur in children younger than 5 years of age, the proportion of DALYs incurred during childhood fell accordingly. A smaller, but still noteworthy decrease (27%) in DALYs was observed for preterm birth complications, further lowering the DALYs among children.

Other success stories between 1990 and 2010 with respect to the control of leading communicable diseases included measles (80% decline), meningitis (22% decrease), and tuberculosis (19% fall). Malaria was an exception to this pattern, with a 20% increase in DALYs between 1990 and 2010.

The rise of noncommunicable diseases as contributors to DALYs between 1990 and 2010 was particularly striking for diabetes (69%), low back pain (43%), depression (38%), ischemic heart disease (29%), and stroke (19%).

Regional differences in the composition of DALYs in 2010 were substantial, with about half of the totals in the high income regions of Asia, Western Europe, Australasia, and North America related to disabilities compared with only about one fifth of the DALYs in the low-income region of sub-Saharan Africa. The underlying causes differed strikingly as well: in the high-income regions, communicable, maternal, neonatal, and nutritional disorders contributed 7% of DALYs, but these same conditions constituted more than two thirds of all DALYs in sub-Saharan Africa.

Risk Factors

The investigators of the GBD 2010 study attempted to characterize the underlying risk factors contributing to the burden of disease globally. The process of estimating the impact of an individual risk factor required multiple elements:

1. Locating data on population exposure to the risk factor.

2. Obtaining sufficient prior research that could be used to define strengths of associations between the risk factors and disease outcomes, as well as support for casual inferences.

3. Determining that the relationships observed between the risk factor and outcome were generalizable to populations other than the ones in which the associations were established.

The disease burden contributions of individual risk factors were assessed against a baseline level; no exposure when possible (i.e., tobacco smoking) or when not possible (i.e., systolic blood pressure), against a minimum risk of exposure level that was supported by epidemiologic evidence and was theoretically possible in a population. The investigators quantified the burden of disease in terms of deaths and separately in DALYs. For simplicity, only the analyses in relation to DALYs are summarized here. A total of 67 individual risk factors and clusters of risk factors were considered in this study.

The 10 leading factors in terms of contributions to DALYs in 2010 are shown in Table 3-4. Elevated blood pressure had the greatest impact on burden of disease followed by tobacco smoking and household pollution from the use of solid fuels. Childhood underweight was the only one of the top 10 risk factors that did not relate to the risk of chronic, degenerative disease. The global decline in the burden from communicable, maternal, neonatal, and nutritional diseases was associated with a corresponding fall in contribution of the risk factors for these conditions. In 1990, childhood underweight was the risk factor with the greatest global disease burden, but it fell to number 8 by 2010. Similarly, suboptimal breastfeeding fell from the fifth highest risk factor contribution in 1990 to 14th in 2010. Other risk factors that declined appreciably in impact on disease burden over those two decades were sanitation (15th to 26th), vitamin A deficiency (17th to 29th), zinc deficiency (19th to 31st), and unimproved water (22nd to 34th). The risk factors that gained the most in terms of contribution to global burden of disease during this time interval were high blood pressure (4th position to 1st), low fruit consumption (7th to 4th), alcohol use (8th to 5th), high body mass index (BMI) (10th to 6th), and drug use (25th to 19th).

There were many parallels between males and females for leading risk factors, with a few key differences. Tobacco smoking was the leading risk factor for males, accounting for 8.4% of DALYs. Among females, however, tobacco smoking was ranked fourth and was responsible for only 3.7% of DALYs. Alcohol use was the third highest risk factor among males, corresponding to 5.4% of DALYs. In contrast, for females, alcohol use was the 12th highest risk factor, accounting for only 2% of DALYs. In contrast, iron deficiency ranked 10th among risk factors for females and contributed

to more than 2% of DALYs. For males, iron deficiency ranked 18th and was responsible for less than 1% of DALYs. Similarly, intimate partner violence was ranked 16th for females at 1.5% of DALYs but was not quantified for males.

Table 3-4 Burden of disease contributions of the 10 leading risk factors, as measured by percentage of global disability-adjusted life years (DALYs) in 2010

Risk Factor	Percent of DALYs
High blood pressure	7.0
Tobacco smoking	6.3
Household air pollution from solid fuels	4.3
Diet low in fruits	4.2
Alcohol use	3.9
High body mass index	3.8
High fasting plasma glucose	3.6
Childhood underweight	3.1
Ambient particulate air pollution	3.1
Physical inactivity	2.8

Data from Lim SS, Vos T, Flaxman AD, et al. A comparative risk assessment of burden of disease and injury attributable to 67 risk factor clusters in 21 regions, 1990-2010: a systematic analysis for the Global Burden of Disease Study 2010. *Lancet.* 2012;380:2224-2260.

Not surprisingly, considerable differences were observed across regions in the relative contributions of various risk factors. For example, childhood underweight, household air pollution from solid fuels, suboptimal breastfeeding, and iron deficiency were the top four risk factors in Eastern, Central, and Western sub-Saharan Africa. Alcohol use was the leading risk factor in three regions: Eastern Europe, Andean Latin America, and Southern sub-Saharan Africa. High BMI was the leading risk factor in Australasia, Southern and Central Latin America, whereas it made a comparatively smaller contribution in Asia and sub-Saharan Africa. Physical inactivity played a greater role in the high-income regions of Asia, Western Europe, Australasia, and North America than in most other parts of the world.

SUMMARY

In this chapter, we have reported key findings about

global health from one of the most comprehensive assessments ever undertaken, the GBD Study of 2010. Key results included:

1. An estimated 52.8 million deaths occurred in 2010.

2. Compared with 1990, a greater number of deaths occurred in 2010 despite lower age-specific death rates because the world's population had grown and aged in the interim.

3. The leading cause of death worldwide was ischemic heart disease, and the three top causes of death all were noncommunicable diseases.

4. The greatest declines in age-standardized mortality rates were for three communicable diseases, measles, diarrheal diseases, and tuberculosis.

5. The observed decline of mortality from infectious disease in developing countries resulting from improved sanitation, nutrition, immunization, and medical care with consequent rises in noncommunicable diseases and growth and aging of the population is referred to as the epidemiologic transition.

6. Between 1990 and 2010, the global life expectancy at birth grew almost 5 years to 67.5 in males and more than 5 years to 73.3 in females.

7. In 2010, the shortest life expectancies were observed in Haiti, largely driven by the devastating earthquake there, and in sub-Saharan Africa because of HIV/AIDS.

8. In 2010, the longest life expectancies were found in the high-income regions of Asia and Western Europe.

9. In 2010, the global healthy life expectancy was 59.0 years for males and 63.2 years for females.

10. DALYs were used as a global measure of disease burden, combining information on both premature deaths and years lived with disability.

11. In 2010, there were 2.5 billion DALYs calculated for the world, with premature deaths accounting for about two thirds of the disease burden, although a shift over time to a greater contribution from disabilities was observed.

12. In 2010, more than half of all global DALYs related to noncommunicable diseases, with another third associated with communicable, maternal, neo-

natal, and nutritional deficiency conditions and the remainder attributable to injuries.

13. Cancer, heart disease, and lower respiratory infections were the three leading causes of loss of healthy life in 2010.

14. Over time, the global burden of disease has shifted from children younger than 5 years of age, although in sub-Saharan Africa, communicable, maternal, neonatal, and nutritional deficiency diseases still account for two thirds of loss of healthy life.

15. The top three risk factors contributing to premature death and disability globally in 2010 were elevated blood pressure, tobacco smoking, and household air pollution from the use of solid fuels.

(Na He)

IMPORTANT TERMINOLOGY

burden of diseases	疾病负担
global burden of diseases	全球疾病负担
morbidity	发病率
mortality	死亡率
life expectancy	期望寿命
healthy life expectancy	健康期望寿命
disability	伤残／失能
disability-adjusted life years	伤残调整生命年
assessment	评估
risk factors	危险因素

 STUDY QUESTIONS

1. Which of the following is NOT associated with the epidemiologic transition?

A. Aging of the population

B. A decline in infectious diseases

C. Growth of the population

D. A decline in noncommunicable diseases

E. Improved sanitation, nutrition and medical care

2. Worldwide, the leading cause of death in 2010 was

A. HIV/AIDS.

B. ischemic heart disease.

C. diarrheal disease.

D. stroke.

E. cancer.

3. *Between 1990 and 2010, the greatest percentage decline in age-standardized mortality rates was found from which disease?*

    A. *Ischemic heart disease*

    B. *Stroke*

    C. *Measles*

    D. *HIV/AIDS*

    E. *Preterm mortality*

4. *The greatest percentage contribution to global burden of disease in 2010, as measured by DALYs, relates to which of the following?*

    A. *Communicable diseases*

    B. *Noncommunicable diseases*

    C. *Injuries*

    D. *Neonatal diseases*

    E. *Elevated blood pressure*

5. *DALYs include consideration of the impact from which of the following?*

    A. *Premature mortality*

    B. *Disability*

    C. *Both premature mortality and disability*

    D. *Neither premature mortality nor disability*

    E. *None of the above*

FURTHER READING

Are C, Rajaram S, Are M, et al. A review of global cancer burden: trends, challenges, strategies, and a role for surgeons. *J Surg Oncol.* 2013;107:221-226.

Eaton J, McCay L, Semrau M, et al. Scale up of services for mental health in low-income and middle-income countries. *Lancet.* 2011;378:1592-1603.

Friel S, Bowen K, Campbell-Lendrum D, Frumkin H, McMichael AJ, Rasanathan K. Climate change, noncommunicable disease, and development: the relationships and common policy opportunities. *Annu Rev Public Health.* 2011;32:133-147.

Gaziano TA, Bitton A, Anand S, Abrahams-Gessel S, Murphy A. Growing epidemic of coronary heart disease in low-and middle income countries. *Curr Probl Cardiol.* 2010;35:72-115.

Harper K, Armelagos G. The changing disease-scape in the Third Epidemiological Transition. *Int J Environ Res Public Health.* 2010;7:675-697.

Kohl HW 3rd, Craig CL, Lambert EV, et al. Lancet Physical Activity Series Working Group. The pandemic of physical inactivity: global action for public health. *Lancet.* 2012;380:294-305.

Malik VS, Willett WC, Hu FB. Global obesity: trends, risk factors and policy implications. *Nat Rev Endocrinol.* 2013;9:12-27.

Walker CL, Rudan I, Liu L, et al. Global burden of childhood pneumonia and diarrhea. *Lancet.* 2013;381:1405-1416.

REFERENCES

GBD 2010

Das P, Samarasekera U. The story of GBD 2010: a "superhuman" effort. *Lancet.* 2012;380:2067-2012.

Murray CJL, Ezzati M, Flaxman AD, et al. GBD 2010: design, definitions, and metrics. *Lancet.* 2012;380:2063-2066.

Mortality

Lozano R, Pourmalek F, Raju M, et al. Global and regional mortality from 235 causes of death for 20 age groups in 1990 and 2010: a systematic analysis for the Global Burden of Disease Study 2010. *Lancet.* 2012;380:2095-2128.

Life Expectancy

Wang H, Dwyer-Lindgren L, Lofgren KT, et al. Age-specific and sex-specific mortality in 187 countries, 1970-2010: a systematic analysis for the Global Burden of Disease Study 2010. *Lancet.* 2012;380:2071-2094.

Healthy Life Expectancy

Salomon JA, Wang H, Freeman MK, et al. Healthy life expectancy for 187 countries, 1990-2010: a systematic analysis for the Global Burden of Disease Study 2010. *Lancet.* 2012; 380:2144-2162.

Disability-Adjusted Life Years

Murray CJL, Vos T, Lozano R, et al. Disability-adjusted life years (DALYs) for 291 diseases and injuries in 21 regions, 1990-2010: a systematic analysis for the Global Burden of Disease Study 2010. *Lancet.* 2012;380:2197-2223.

Risk Factors

Lim SS, Vos T, Flaxman AD, et al. A comparative risk assessment of burden of disease and injury attributable to 67 risk factor clusters in 21 regions, 1990-2010: a systematic analysis for the Global Burden of Disease Study 2010. *Lancet.* 2012;380:2224-2260.

Descriptive Epidemiology

4

HEALTH SCENARIO

A 62-year-old healthy female office manager with fair skin visited her dermatologist for the evaluation of a recently appearing itchy black mole on her left thigh. Upon examination, the mole was approximately 8 mm in diameter with an asymmetrical shape, irregular borders, black and brown coloration, and a flat surface. An excisional biopsy with 1cm surgical margins was performed revealing a superficial spreading melanoma of 0.6-mm thickness without ulceration or evidence of rapid cell division. There was no disease spread beyond the primary anatomic site, and the patient was followed with regular examinations, which revealed no recurrence or spread during the following 5 years.

CLINICAL BACKGROUND

Melanoma is a malignancy of pigment-producing cells (melanocytes) principally found in the skin. It is the fifth most common form of cancer in the United States, with more than 75,000 cases diagnosed each year. Although fewer than 5% of skin cancers are melanomas, four out of five deaths from skin cancer are related to melanoma.

Melanomas typically present, as in the patient described, as non-uniform pigmented skin lesions that have changed over time. The lesions may have shades of brown, black, red, or blue discoloration. The appearance usually is asymmetrical, and the boundaries are often indistinct or irregular. At diagnosis, the size usually exceeds a half centimeter.

Melanoma occurs much more frequently among whites than among those of other races. It tends to

arise more frequently in older persons but can occur as early as the second or third decades of life. Fair-skinned persons, as in the patient described earlier, are at increased risk as are those with light hair color, blue eyes, and a predisposition to freckling.

Persons with a family history of melanoma are at increased risk, and a number of genes have been associated with a predisposition to developing this disease. Persons who have had a previous melanoma are at greatly elevated risk of developing a second melanoma. By far, the strongest environmental risk factor for this disease is exposure to ultraviolet (UV) radiation. This can occur through sunlight exposure, as demonstrated by cumulative indices of exposure, as well as frequency of sunburn events. The use of tanning beds also has been linked to melanoma risk, especially among young adults who are regular users.

A diagnosis of melanoma is confirmed by a surgical biopsy that removes some or all of the lesion for microscopic examination by a pathologist. There are five subtypes of melanoma, with about two thirds classified as the superficial spreading type. These cancers begin as a proliferation of melanocytes in the basal layer of the skin and tend to grow by radial (outward) expansion followed eventually by vertical (upward) expansion.

Several microscopic features have been shown to be related to the prognosis of melanomas. One of the most important attributes is the vertical penetration of the lesion, with tumors divided into thin (<1 mm), intermediate (1–4 mm), and thick (>4 mm) levels. Patients with thinner melanomas tend to have better clinical outcomes. Other attributes that affect prognosis are ulceration (loss of the overlying epithelium), which is associated with worse prognosis, and mitotic activity, with higher levels of cell reproduction being linked to poorer outcomes.

The primary treatment for cutaneous melanoma is surgical removal. It is important that the entire malignancy be removed, as evidenced by margins that lack cancer cells. The recommended width of the clear margins depends on the size of the tumor. For the majority of patients with thin, non-ulcerated, low mitotic rate tumors, as in our example, no further evaluation generally is required. For those with adverse prognosis factors, however, imaging studies or sampling of lymph nodes (or both) may be indicated to determine whether the cancer has spread to regional lymph nodes or beyond. For patients with high-risk or advanced disease, interferon is the only treatment shown to slow the spread of disease and improve overall survival. Interferon is a glycoprotein that binds to a specific membrane receptor, leading to the activation of genes that produce substances that interfere with cancer growth by inhibiting cell proliferation and preventing the growth of new blood vessels to nourish the tumor. Other systemic treatments for disseminated melanoma are under evaluation.

DESCRIPTIVE EPIDEMIOLOGY

In Chapter 1, we learned that one of the primary uses of epidemiology is descriptive, by which we mean evaluation of the distribution of a disease within a population. We contrasted this application with analytic epidemiology, which focuses on the study of potential causes of a disease.

These two types of epidemiology each serve essential purposes and may be seen as complementary in nature. Descriptive studies often lead to speculation about underlying patterns of occurrence and why some population groups appear to be at higher (or lower) risk of becoming affected. These theories could be tested in a subsequent analytic study. Similarly, analytic studies may shed light on reasons for variation in disease occurrence within populations, leading to more focused surveillance strategies.

In this chapter, we focus on **descriptive epidemiology**, using malignant melanoma as the illustrative example. Descriptive studies can be used to assess the burden of a disease in a community, but also to investigate possible correlations, surveil health status in the population or community, study disease clustering, and monitor the effectiveness of health interventions.

For this purpose, we will use the tools of measurement that were introduced in Chapter 2, including the incidence, prevalence, and mortality. We are guided in this effort by three basic questions of descriptive epidemiology:

1. Who develops the disease (melanoma)?

2. Where does the disease (melanoma) tend to occur?

3. When does the disease (melanoma) tend to occur?

In answering these questions, we characterize the distribution of melanoma by person, place, and time. We can think of these three dimensions as helping us to map out the population distribution of melanoma, as depicted schematically in Figure 4-1.

PERSON

As noted in Chapter 1, one of the fundamental tenets of epidemiology is that diseases do not occur at random. In other words, some people, by virtue of their personal characteristics, have a heightened risk of developing the disease. Other persons, by virtue of their own attributes, have a lowered risk of the disease. The job of the epidemiologist is to ascertain which of these personal attributes is most highly associated with risk.

The most basic place to begin with is demographic characteristics such as age, race, and sex. This information is available routinely from clinical and other sources of information on the affected individuals, as well as on the population from which they arose.

The incidence of melanoma in the United States is shown by age in Figure 4-2. Incidence data are available for cancer in the United States through a variety of mechanisms. One is the Surveillance,

Epidemiology and End Results (SEER) Program of the National Cancer Institute. The SEER Program, created in 1973, involves a network of cancer registries that collectively cover more than one quarter of the U.S. population. A disease registry is an organized system for collecting information on persons with a disease of interest. Registries can be hospital based, meaning that they focus on patients treated at a specific health care facility or group of facilities. Other registries are population based, meaning that an attempt is made to collect information on all affected persons who reside within a particular area. The SEER registry system is population based and involves 20 areas selected to be broadly representative of the United States.

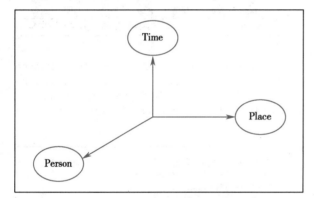

Figure 4-1. Schematic representation of the standard dimensions used to characterize disease occurrence.

A second population-based cancer registration system in the United States is the National Program of Cancer Registries, first organized in 1992 and coordinated by the Centers for Disease Control and Prevention (CDC). Today, this program includes data from 45 states and territories, which correspond to 96% of the U.S. population. The data presented in Figure 4-2 were derived from the SEER Program. We can see that melanoma is a strongly age-dependent condition, with a dramatic rise in incidence with age. In general, cancer is a disease that tends to predominate at older ages.

The incidence of melanoma is depicted by race and ethnicity in Figure 4-3. There is a dramatic differential, with the highest risk among non-Hispanic whites and the lowest risks among Asians and blacks. 20 to 30 fold difference in risk across race/ethnic groups is highly unusual and is therefore an important clue to the underlying risk factors. One possible explanation for this pattern is that darker, more pigmented skin tends to protect against the damage caused by UV radiation. Other factors related to European ancestry may be involved as well, including genetic susceptibility.

The incidence of melanoma by sex is illustrated in Figure 4-4. Here we see a 60% excess of disease among males. These summary results are heavily reflective of the pattern among non-Hispanic whites because that particular race/ethnic group so dominates the overall occurrence patterns. A male excess is seen in some, but not all, race/ethnic groups in the United States and elsewhere, so there may be factors related to sunlight exposure patterns or other risk factors that explain this disparity.

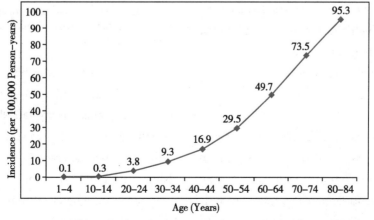

Figure 4-2. Incidence rates for melanoma, by age, United States, 2006 to 2010. (Data from Howlader N, et al. SEER Cancer Statistics Review, 1975-2010. Bethesda, MD: National Cancer Institute; 2013.)

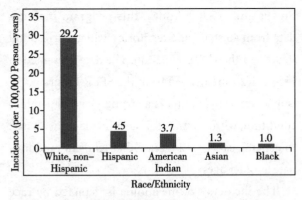

Figure 4-3. Incidence rates of melanoma, by race/ethnicity, in the United States, 2006 to 2010. (Data from Howlader N, et al. SEER Cancer Statistics Review, 1975-2010. Bethesda, MD: National Cancer Institute; 2013.)

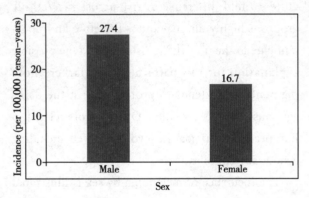

Figure 4-4. Incidence rates for melanoma, by sex, United States, 2006 to 2010. (Data from Howlader N, et al. SEER Cancer Statistics Review, 1975-2010. Bethesda, MD: National Cancer Institute; 2013.)

It is also worth noting that the male excess of melanoma in the United States appears principally at older ages. As illustrated in Figure 4-5, there is a progressive increase in the male-to-female ratio of melanoma incidence with age. Before age 50 years, females exhibit excesses of the disease, with male excesses occurring over age 50 years. It has been speculated that the high risk among young women may relate to more frequent UV radiation exposure by sunlight, use of tanning beds, or both.

PLACE

Variation in disease occurrence by place of residence can be examined across countries or within them. In Figure 4-6, incidence rates for melanoma among men are shown for representative countries of residence. Tremendous variation is seen, with the highest rates in the Oceanic region (Australia and New Zea-

land) and the lowest rates in Asia. (African countries were not included here because of extremely low rates and poor registration systems.) North American and Northern European countries tend to have moderately high rates, with lower rates in Southern Europe and South America. The corresponding incidence patterns for females are shown in Figure 4-7, with similar rankings, except for Denmark replacing the United States with the second highest rates.

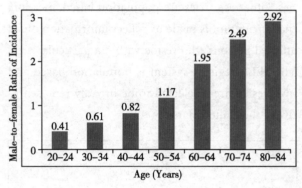

Figure 4-5. Male-to-female ratio of melanoma incidence among whites, by age, United States, 2008 to 2010. (Data from Howlader N, et al. SEER Cancer Statistics Review, 1975-2010. Bethesda, MD: National Cancer Institute; 2013.)

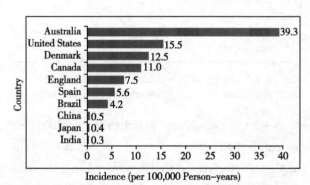

Figure 4-6. Incidence rates for melanoma, by country, for males, 2000 to 2002. (Data from Erdman F et al. International trends in the incidence of malignant melanoma 1953-2008: are recent generations at higher or lower risk? Int J Cancer. 2013;132:385-400.)

These patterns of international variation in the disease incidence tend to support the general notion of elevated rates among fair-skinned populations (Northern Europe, North America, and Oceania). Within Europe, the gradient of increasing rates with rising latitude is consistent with a gradient in skin pigmentation. The combination of fair skin and heavy sunlight exposure, as occurs in Oceania, results in the highest overall risk of melanoma.

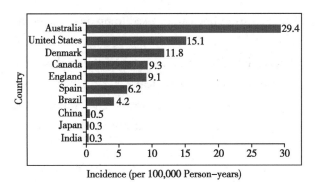

Figure 4-7. Incidence rates for melanoma, by country, for females, 2000 to 2002. (Data from Erdman F et al. International trends in the incidence of malignant melanoma 1953-2008: are recent generations at higher or lower risk? Int J Cancer. 2013;132:385-400.)

Variation in disease occurrence also can be examined by place of residence within a single country. One such analysis was performed in Norway, a country with a homogeneous, fair-skinned population. Overall, Norway is located at high latitude, but it extends across a considerable geographic range (57–72° N), allowing a comparison of incidence in the northern and southern parts of the country. The rates in the south of Norway are twice the corresponding rates in the north of the country, consistent with the greater sunlight exposure in the south.

CORRELATIONS WITH DISEASE OCCURRENCE

The variation of disease occurrence patterns across population groups can be used to generate hypotheses about the reasons for this variation. Such a study may be useful for suggesting potential risk factors for the disease because it is relatively quick, inexpensive, and easy to perform. This type of investigation is referred to as an ecologic study because it examines the pattern of risk at the group or population level rather than on a person-by-person basis. Such a study might also be referred to as a correlation study because it results in a measure of how strongly disease occurrence is related to some potentially predictive characteristics.

To illustrate an ecologic study, data are presented in Figure 4-8 on the mortality rate of melanoma in relation to the annual number of days of

very high UV index, a measure of intensity of UV radiation from the sun. For this analysis, eight Midwestern states were chosen because they have stable populations and are relatively homogeneous with respect to race and ethnicity. The states included were North Dakota, South Dakota, Minnesota, Iowa, Nebraska, Missouri, Kansas, and Oklahoma. Mortality rates were used here rather than incidence rates because the former was readily available for all states. The UV index data were from a period more than a decade before the mortality experience, thereby accounting for a lag in time from exposure to the development of disease and subsequent clinical course. An even longer lag period might have been justified given the presumed length of exposure required for melanoma to develop, but earlier measures of UV index were not universally available.

The scatter plot in Figure 4-8 reveals a generally positive relationship between days of very high UV index and mortality from melanoma, with states with more days of intense sunlight exposure (e.g., Oklahoma and Kansas) experiencing higher rates of death from melanoma. In contrast, states with fewer days of intense solar radiation (e.g., North Dakota and Minnesota) had lower rates of death from melanoma.

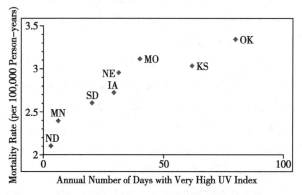

Figure 4-8. Scatterplot of mortality rate of melanoma (2006–2010) in relation to annual days of very high ultraviolet index (1995) for eight selected states in the Midwestern United States. (Melanoma data from Howlader N, et al. SEER Cancer Statistics Review, 1975-2010. Bethesda, MD: National Cancer Institute; 2013. UV index data from Climate Prediction Center, National Weather Service, National Oceanic and Atmospheric Administration: UV Index: Annual Time Series. College Park, MD; 2013.)

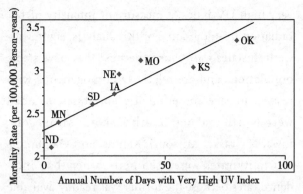

Figure 4-9. Regression line for regression of mortality from melanoma (2006–2010) on annual days of very high ultraviolet index (1995). (Melanoma data from Howlader N, et al. SEER Cancer Statistics Review, 1975-2010. Bethesda, MD: National Cancer Institute; 2013. UV index data from Climate Prediction Center, National Weather Service, National Oceanic and Atmospheric Administration: UV Index: Annual Time Series. College Park, MD; 2013.)

To assess the strengths of relationships between days of very high UV index and death rate from melanoma, a **correlation analysis** was performed on these data. If very high UV index and melanoma mortality were maximally correlated, the correlation coefficient would be 1.0. If there was no relationship at all, then the correlation coefficient would be zero. If there was a maximally inverse relationship (i.e., melanoma deaths tended to occur more frequently in areas with lower UV index), the correlation coefficient would be-1.0. The calculated correlation coefficient was 0.91, which confirms the visual impression that the measure of intense solar radiation and melanoma death rates are strongly and positively linked.

The square of the correlation coefficient is 0.83, and this is referred to as the coefficient of determination. An interpretation of this finding is that more than four fifths of the variation observed in melanoma mortality rates can be accounted for by the number of days of very high UV index.

A linear regression analysis of these data revealed the following equation:

$$\text{Mortality} = 2.30 + 0.014(\text{Days UV index})$$

A graph of this regression line is shown in Figure 4-9. This relationship is highly statistically significant, meaning that it is very unlikely that the observed relationship could have occurred by chance alone.

The regression line can be used to predict melanoma mortality. For instance, in the absence of any days of very high UV index, the predicted mortality from melanoma would be 2.30 deaths per 100,000 person-years. For every 10 days of very high UV index, the death rate increases 0.14 deaths per 100,000 person-years.

As shown visually and by regression analysis, the relationship between intense solar UV radiation and risk of melanoma death is very strong, raising the question of whether intense solar UV radiation might be a cause of melanoma. Unfortunately, this type of ecologic study cannot prove whether an association arises from a causal link. The observations are at the group (state) level of experience, so we do not know what is happening at the individual person level. Although the overall group risk of melanoma death is higher for populations living in areas with more intense sun exposure, the persons who developed melanoma in these communities may have less solar exposure because they have fair skin and burn easily. Epidemiologists refer to this type of inconsistency as an ecologic fallacy. That is to say, at the group level, a risk factor and a disease appear to be tightly linked, but at the personal level, there is no such association.

Given the potential for an ecologic fallacy, one might wonder why such a study would be undertaken in the first place. The motivation for conducting an ecologic study is that it relies on easily accessible already collected data. It is quick and inexpensive, therefore, to conduct such an investigation compared with the more definitive types of study on individual subjects. This type of "quick and dirty" study might be used to develop clues or hypotheses about disease causation. We refer to such an investigation as a hypothesis-generating study because its purpose is to develop a theory about disease causation that can be tested subsequently in a more definitive study. These more definitive investigations are more time consuming, complicated, and expensive to conduct, as we will see in later chapters. We refer to these investigations of individual exposure and disease risk as hypothesis-testing studies. Many hypothesis-testing studies have been conducted on personal exposure to solar (and other types of UV) radiation and the risk of melanoma. In general, these investigations have found the most compelling evidence for risk associated with recurrent sunburns in childhood and adolescence.

TIME

The incidence of a disease also can be tracked over time. As shown in Figure 4-10, in the United States, melanoma occurrence has been rising steadily over the years between 1975 and 2010. During this 35-year period of time, the incidence tripled. In recent years, the annual increase has averaged about 2.6%. This pattern is at odds with the experience for cancer of all types, which experienced rising incidence rates until 1992 followed by a progressive decline of about 0.5% per year on average thereafter.

It should be noted that the time trend depicted in Figure 4-10, although representing the experience of the population of the United States, does not correspond to a single, fixed group of people. Over a span of 35 years, the composition of the population evolves as new persons are added by birth and immigration, and other persons are removed by emigration or death.

A slightly different picture might emerge if we were to track the disease occurrence among a group of people born in a particular year or time period (a birth cohort) as they aged through life. For this purpose, it is helpful to have many years of observation, so that multiple successive birth cohorts can be tracked through their lifespans. On a national level, collection of data on cancer occurrence did not start in the United States until the 1970s, but the State of Connecticut has been collecting data on cancer incidence since the 1930s. Data from the Connecticut Tumor Registry are shown in Figure 4-11. For simplicity, age-specific incidence rates are presented for males only and for two time periods. It is clear that there has been a dramatic increase in the occurrence of melanoma between these two data collection periods 30 years apart. The disparity is particularly strong at the age groups above 50 years.

A somewhat different picture emerges if we examine the incidence not by age and time period but rather by age and birth cohort (Figure 4-12). For each successive birth cohort, beginning in 1910 and continuing through 1940, there was a progressively higher incidence of melanoma at each age group. The most recent birth cohort, men born in 1950, however, had age-specific incidence rates that were similar to men born in 1940. Of course, not enough time has elapsed for the men born in 1950 to reach the highest risk years for melanoma. It is possible, therefore, that there may be greater separation of the 1940 and 1950 birth cohorts with regard to melanoma risk at older ages. Nevertheless, from the data available, it appears that there may be a leveling off of melanoma risk for the later birth cohorts of men, suggesting a generational stabilization of exposure to UV radiation.

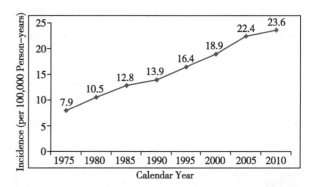

Figure 4-10. Incidence of melanoma, by year, in the United States, 1975 to 2010. (Data from Howlader N, et al. SEER Cancer Statistics Review, 1975-2010. Bethesda, MD: National Cancer Institute; 2013.)

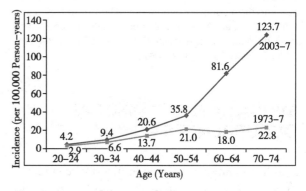

Figure 4-11. Incidence of melanoma among males, by age and time period, Connecticut. (Data from Geller AC, Clapp RW, Sober AJ, et al. Melanoma epidemic: an analysis of six decades of data from the Connecticut Tumor Registry. J ClinOncol. 2013;33:4172-4178.)

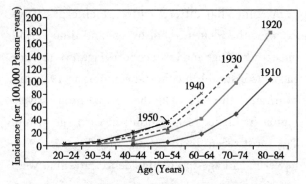

Figure 4-12. Incidence of melanoma among males, by age and birth cohort, Connecticut. (Data from Geller AC, Clapp RW, Sober AJ, et al. Melanoma epidemic: an analysis of six decades of data from the Connecticut Tumor Registry. J ClinOncol. 2013;33:4172-4178.)

It should be noted that the Connecticut data reveal a different pattern for women, with a continued rise in age-specific incidence rates for successive birth cohorts, with no evidence of a plateau (Figure 4-13).

These observations tend to support a continuing generational increase in exposure to UV radiation among females through sunlight, tanning devices, or both.

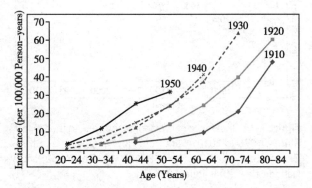

Figure 4-13. Incidence of melanoma among females, by age and birth cohort, Connecticut. (Data from Geller AC, Clapp RW, Sober AJ, et al. Melanoma epidemic: an analysis of six decades of data from the Connecticut Tumor Registry. J ClinOncol. 2013;33:4172-4178.)

MIGRATION AND DISEASE OCCURRENCES

Another technique available in descriptive epidemiology is to examine whether migration affects the rate of disease occurrence. Such a study may help to establish the extent to which a disease is determined by genetic factors, environmental exposures,

or both. Consider, for example, a study in which persons from a country known to be at low risk for a particular disease migrate to a country known to be at high risk for that same disease. If the disease risk among migrants remains low, we might conclude that a change in environment did not affect risk, so that disease susceptibility is either established by heredity or premigration environmental exposure. If we follow disease risk into the next generation, and children of migrants born and raised in the adopted country continue to have a low risk, the reduced risk is transferable across generations and suggests a hereditary basis for the disease.

If, in contrast, migrants from a low-risk country move to a high-risk nation and experience a higher rate of disease than those who did not migrate, we might conclude that environmental exposures do affect risk. In the next generation, as the children of immigrants assimilate into the cultural patterns of the new home country and have a full lifetime of exposure, we would expect disease rates to closely parallel those of native-born persons for conditions that are determined mostly by environmental causes.

A number of migrant studies have been conducted in relation to risk of melanoma. One setting that is especially suited for this type of investigation is Israel, where there are large numbers of immigrants coming from a variety of settings. Investigators in Israel studied melanoma risk among Israeli men of European descent according to when they arrived in Israel. In general, the European countries of origin have much lower incidence rates for melanoma than does Israel. As shown in Figure 4-14, the migrants from Europe who arrived in Israel at 10 years of age or younger experienced risk of melanoma virtually identical to those who were born in Israel. However, migrants from Europe who arrived in Israel at ages older than 10 years had a 40% lower risk of developing melanoma. In other words, environmental exposures early in life appear to be important determinants of risk of malignant melanoma. If one spends the first decade of life in a low-risk setting and then moves to a higher risk country, the relative protection of the low-risk childhood environment appears to persist. The protective effect is lost if one migrates during the first decade of life.

This observation does not establish early childhood sun exposure as a definitive cause of melanoma, but it is consistent with that hypothesis. One cannot exclude other early childhood exposures or hereditary factors from playing some role in causation. Indeed, a number of other lines of investigation support a contribution from genetics to risk of developing melanoma. Nevertheless, it appears that early life experience is important in determining a person's subsequent risk of melanoma.

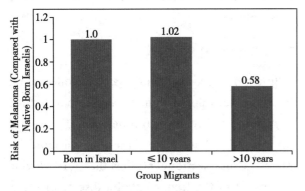

Figure 4-14. Risk of melanoma among Israeli men of European descent, 1967 to 2005, by migrant status and age at migration. (Data from Levine H, Afek A, Shamiss A, et al. Country of origin, age at migration and risk of cutaneous melanoma: a migrant cohort study of 1,100,000 Israeli men. Int J Cancer. 2013;133:486-494.)

MAJOR STUDY DESIGNS AND SOURCES OF DATA

Descriptive epidemiology of a disease pattern can be analyzed from data obtained from various study designs or data sources.

Case Report

Case report is a brief, objective report of a clinical characteristic or outcome from a single clinical subject or event. A case report can address almost any clinical question or issue, including screening test results or treatment outcomes, or natural history findings. It is commonly used to report unusual or unexpected events, such as adverse drug reactions, or previously unrecognized diseases or disease characteristics.

For a case report, a single noteworthy event must be first identified. Data collection is generally retrospective, with a review and a descriptive summary of subjects or events. No statistical analysis or comparison group is included in this type of design. Although few conclusions can be drawn based on evidence from a single event or observation, case reports provide a first report of unexpected findings, which can generate hypotheses for testing, or definitions of issue for further study. The results of a case report are rarely generalizable.

Case Series Report

A case series report is an objective report of a clinical characteristic or outcome from a group of clinical subjects. A case series report can address almost any clinical issue, including screening test results or treatment outcomes and natural history findings. However, it is most commonly used to describe clinical characteristics, such as signs and symptoms of disease, process and quality of the clinical management, or disease outcomes.

In a case series report, subjects must be identified with regard to the clinical events or characteristics in question. Data collection may be retrospective or prospective, but a comparison or control group usually is not included. Descriptive statistics are calculated to define the proportion of subjects with the characteristics under study. Conclusions are generally limited because there is no comparison group within the study. The generalizability of a case series report depends on the representation of the study population. When a consecutive series of subjects, i.e., all eligible subjects are included over a specified period of time can help strengthen the study results.

Clinical Data Registry

A clinical data registry is a special case of the case series report, which records information about the health status of patients and the health care they receive over varying periods of time. Clinical data registries typically focus on patients who share a common reason for needing health care. They allow health care professionals and others to see what treatments are available, and how patients with different characteristics respond to various treatments. This information can be used to inform patients and their health care professionals as they decide the best course of treatment and to improve care for patients in the future. Information from registries may also be used to compare the performance of healthcare providers with regard to their outcomes and resource use.

There are many types of clinical data registries including those that focus on a disease or condition (e.g., cystic fibrosis), a procedure (e.g., coronary artery bypass grafting surgery) or to track the performance of a device (e.g. artificial joint). A clinical data registry begins by defining a patient population, and then recruits health care professionals who will submit data on a representative sample of these patients. For each patient population, a variety of treatments may be available. By studying many aspects of the populations patterns associated with particular outcomes can be identified. Since all of the factors that might have an impact on outcomes are not necessarily known at the time of data collection, data can be stored for use at a later time to evaluate previously unrecognized associations.

Patients often receive care from different organizations over time. Each time a patient participating in a registry sees their health care professional or is admitted to a hospital, detailed data are recorded about their health status and the care received. Health care professionals then send encrypted data about the patients to the clinical data registry through a highly secure web portal or from their electronic health record. As data enters the clinical data registry, quality checks are performed to ensure the correctness and completeness of the data. If something is missing or outside of the expected range, registry staff contact the submitting health care professional asking them to review and verify the data.

Clinical data registries provide information to health care professionals to improve the quality and safety of the care they provide to their patients. For example, the use of evidence-based practice

guidelines can be evaluated by asking questions like, "How many patients are receiving recommended treatment(s)?" In addition, information from clinical data registries is used to compare the effectiveness of different treatments for the same disease or condition, to evaluate different approaches to a procedure and to monitor the safety of implanted devices. The information from clinical data registries is also used to support health care education, accreditation and certification. Finally, information from clinical data registries is increasingly used to ensure that payment is adjusted based on the quality of care provided and to give patients the information they need to make better choices.

Cross-Sectional Studies

In a cross-sectional study, data are collected on the whole study population at a single point in time to examine the relationship between disease (or other health related state) and other variables of interest. **Cross-sectional studies** therefore provide a snapshot of the frequency of a disease or other health related characteristics in a population at a given point in time. This methodology can be used to assess the burden of disease or health needs of a population, for example, and is therefore particularly useful in informing the planning and allocation of health resources.

A cross-sectional study may be purely descriptive and used to assess the frequency and distribution of a particular disease in a defined population. For example, a random sample of schools across London may be used to assess the burden or prevalence of asthma among 12-14 year olds.

Analytical cross-sectional studies may also be used to investigate the association between a putative risk factor and a health outcome. However, this type of study is limited in its ability to draw valid conclusions about any association or possible causality because the presence of risk factors and outcomes are measured simultaneously. It may therefore be difficult to work out whether the disease or the exposure came first, so causation should always be confirmed by more rigorous studies. The collection of information about risk factors is also retrospective, running the risk of recall bias. In practice cross-sectional studies will include an element of both types of design.

A cross-sectional study should be representative of the whole population, if generalizations from the findings are to have any validity. For example, a study of the prevalence of diabetes among women aged 40-60 years in Town A should comprise a random sample of all women aged 40-60 years in that town. If the study is to be representative, attempts should be made to include hard to reach groups, such as people in institutions or the homeless.

The sample size should be sufficiently large enough to estimate the prevalence of the conditions of interest with adequate precision. Sample size calculations can be carried out using sample size tables or statistical packages. The larger the study, the less likely the results are due to chance alone, but this will also have implications for cost.

As data on exposures and outcomes are collected simultaneously, specific inclusion and exclusion criteria should be established at the design stage, to ensure that those with the outcome are correctly identified. The data collection methods will depend on the exposure, outcome and study setting, but include questionnaires and interviews, as well as medical examinations. Routine data sources may also be used.

Non-response is a particular problem affecting cross-sectional studies and can result in bias of the measures of outcome. This is a particular problem when the characteristics of non-responders differ from responders.

In a cross-sectional study all factors (exposure, outcome, and confounders) are measured simultaneously. The main outcome measure obtained from a cross-sectional study is prevalence. For continuous variables such as blood pressure or weight, values will fall along a continuum within a given range. Prevalence may therefore only be calculated when the variable is divided into those values that fall below or above a particular pre-determined level. Alternatively mean or median levels may be calculated.

In analytical cross-sectional studies the odds ratio can be used to assess the strength of an association between a risk factor and health outcome of interest, providing that the current exposure accurately reflects the past exposure.

Cross-sectional studies have several major strengths. They are relatively quick and easy to conduct with no long periods of follow-up and data on all variables is only collected once. The study design allows for measuring prevalence for all factors under investigation and multiple outcomes and exposures can be studied. The major weaknesses of such a design include the difficulty to determine whether the outcome followed exposure in time or exposure resulted from the outcome, thus an associations identified may be difficult to interpret. Such a design is also susceptible to bias due to low response and misclassification due to recall bias.

Ecological Studies

Ecological studies, or geographical studies, can be used to demonstrate patterns of disease and associated factors at population level, but not at individual level. The units of study are populations or groups. As presented in the previous section "Correlation with Disease Occurrence", results are mainly from ecological studies.

This type of study can be used to generate hypotheses of possible causes or determinants of disease, for example if broad geographical differences are seen, but cannot be used to prove this or explore associations in any depth. Further observational or even interventional studies are needed to do this.

Ecological studies usually make use of routinely collected health information, so their principal advantage is that they are cheap and quick to complete. Ecological studies can also utilize geographical information systems to examine spatial framework of disease and exposure. However, the appropriate data may not be readily available and in these circumstances it is necessary to carry out special surveys to collect the raw material necessary for the study.

In such a design, measures of exposure are only a proxy based on the average in the population, thus caution is needed when applying grouped results to the individual level (**ecological fallacy**). The ecological fallacy is an error in the interpretation of statistical data in an ecological study when conclusions are made about individuals from the aggregated data inappropriately. The fallacy assumes that all members of a group have the average characteristics of the group as whole, when in fact any association observed between variables at the group level does not necessarily mean that the same association exists for an individual plucked from the group. Reasons for the ecological fallacy include:

- It is not possible to link exposure with disease in individuals —those with disease may not be the same people in the population who are exposed;
- Data used in descriptive studies were usually collected for other purposes originally;
- Use of average exposure levels may mask more complicated relationships with the disease;
- Inability to control for confounding.

SUMMARY

In this chapter, the methods of descriptive epidemiology were illustrated with data on the occurrence of melanoma. Fundamental to descriptive epidemiology is the premise that diseases do not occur at random. Some persons, by virtue of their personal characteristics, are at increased risk of the disease, and other persons are at reduced risk of being affected. These patterns often are revealed by answers to three basic questions:

1. Who gets the disease?
2. Where does the disease occur?
3. When does the disease occur?

These features of disease occurrence relate respectively to person, place and time.

The standard approach to characterizing who gets the disease begins with demographic attributes such as age, race, and sex. For melanoma, we observed that the disease occurs with increased frequency in older persons, white non-Hispanics, and males.

The place of occurrence can be evaluated on the international, national, or regional levels. For melanoma, the greatest incidence rates tend to occur in Oceania followed by North America and northern Europe. Within some countries, gradients of risk by geographic latitude also are observed.

Unlike cancer overall in developed countries, the incidence of melanoma is increasing over time, with more than a 2% per year increase in the United States. When 6 decades of data from Connecticut were examined by birth cohort, that is, by groups born in the same year or period, increasing incidence appears to apply to successive birth years for both males and females up until 1950. Thereafter, a leveling off was observed among males, and continuing generational increases were seen for females.

Ecologic studies can be conducted to correlate the group level exposure to a putative causative agent with the occurrence of disease. We illustrated this approach with data from eight states in the Midwestern United States concerning annual number of days with very high UV index and subsequent mortality rates for melanoma. Although a strong correlation was demonstrated, the absence of data at the individual subject level prevents one from concluding that heavily UV-exposed persons bear an increased risk of melanoma. An ecologic fallacy exists when an exposure and disease appear to be linked at the population level but not within specific individuals.

We considered how investigation of migrant populations can help to distinguish whether a disease is primarily determined by inherited traits or is more greatly influenced by environmental exposures. An illustrative study was cited in which migrants from Europe to Israel had incident rates of melanoma similar to native-born Israelis if they migrated within the first decade of life. If they migrated later, however, they tended to retain risks of melanoma that were more similar to those of their European countries of origin. These findings tend to support the notion that environmental exposures early in life are particularly critical in determining the risk of melanoma later in life.

Data from major study designs, such as case report, case series report, clinical registry, cross-sectional study, and ecological study can be used for descriptive analysis of disease occurrence. The strengths and weaknesses of each study design should be considered when such a design is used.

(**Zhijie Zheng**)

IMPORTANT TERMINOLOGY

descriptive epidemiology	描述性流行病学
correlation analysis	相关分析
cross-sectional studies	横断面研究
ecological studies	生态学研究
ecological fallacy	生态学谬误

 STUDY QUESTIONS

1. *Which of the following attributes is NOT typically used to characterize who gets a disease?*

    A. *Sex*

    B. *HLA type*

    C. *Race*

    D. *Age*

2. *Persons born in the same year are referred to as*

    A. *a birth cohort.*

    B. *gestational peers.*

    C. *conception cohort.*

    D. *none of the above.*

3. *For a genetic disease, when persons from a high-risk country migrate to a low-risk country, we expect their risk of disease to*

    A. *decrease.*

    B. *increase.*

    C. *remain unchanged.*

    D. *vary based on age at migration.*

4. *For an environmentally determined disease, when persons migrate from a high-risk country to a low-risk country, we expect their risk of disease to*

    A. *decrease.*

    B. *increase.*

    C. *remain unchanged.*

    D. *be similar to their children's risk.*

5. *In an ecologic study of cell phone use and incidence of brain cancer, the coefficient of determination is found to be 0.3. This suggests that*

    A. *cell phone use accounts for most of the variation in risk of brain cancer.*

    B. *cell phone use is a cause of brain cancer.*

    C. *cell phone use has no association with risk of brain cancer.*

    D. *cell phone use accounts for about a third of the variation in brain cancer risk.*

6. *In an ecologic study of dietary folate intake and risk of neural tube defects, the correlation coefficient was-0.86. This means that*

    A. *high dietary folate intake is associated with a higher risk of neural tube defects.*

    B. *high dietary folate intake is associated with a lower risk of neural tube defects.*

    C. *there is no association between dietary folate intake and neural tube defects.*

    D. *dietary folate intake causes neural tube defects.*

7. *In a correlation study, the prevalence of obesity is associated at the population level with the incidence of prostate cancer. When examined on a person-by-person basis, however, obese individuals do not have an increased risk of developing prostate cancer. This is an example of*

    A. *the Hawthorne effect.*

    B. *a selection bias.*

    C. *an ecologic fallacy.*

    D. *regression to the mean.*

8. *A registry for Alzheimer's disease is described as population-based. This means that*

    A. *only persons born within a specific population are considered for registration.*

    B. *an attempt is made to assemble a population of Alzheimer's disease patients from specialized treatment centers.*

    C. *only data from population surveys are used to find persons with Alzheimer's disease.*

    D. *an attempt is made to identify all Alzheimer's disease patients from a population defined within geographic boundaries.*

9. *Human papillomavirus (HPV) is known to be the principal cause of uterine cervical cancer. If an ecologic study was performed, one would expect the following correlation coefficient between incidence of HPV cervical infection and incidence of cervical can-*

cer to be closest to

A. −1.

B. 0.

C. 1.

D. 100.

10. Which of the following is NOT a descriptive epidemiology study?

A. A study of trends over time in the mortality from diabetes

B. A study of variation in stroke incidence by race and sex

C. A study of the risk of stomach cancer among migrants

D. A study of the risk of suicide among veterans as compared with nonveterans

FURTHER READING

Gabe C, Leiter U. Melanoma epidemiology and trends. *Clin Dermatol.* 2009;27:3-9.

Little EG, Eide MJ. Update on the current state of melanoma incidence. *Dermatol Clin.* 2012;30:355-361.

Hennekens CH, Buring JE. Epidemiology in Medicine. Lippincott Williams & Wilkins, 1987.

REFERENCES

Clinical Background

Dunki-Jacobs EM, Callender GG, McMasters KM. Current management of melanoma. *CurrProbl Surg.* 2013;50:351-382.

Descriptive Epidemiology

Person

Howlader N, et al. *SEER Cancer Statistics Review, 1975-2010.* Bethesda, MD: National Cancer Institute; 2013.

Place

Cicarma E, Juzeniene A, Porojnicu AC, Bruland ØS, Moan J. Latitude gradient for melanoma incidence by anatomic site and gender in Norway, 1966-2007. *J Photochem Photobiol B.* 2010;101:174-178.

Erdmann F, Lortet-Tieulent J, Schüz J, et al. International trends in the incidence of malignant melanoma, 1953-2008: are recent generations at higher or lower risk? *Int J Cancer.*2013;132:385-400.

Correlations with Disease Occurrence

Climate Prediction Center, National Weather Service, National Oceanic and Atmospheric Administration: *UV Index: Annual Time Series.* College Park, MD: Author; 2013.

Howlader N, et al. *SEER Cancer Statistics Review,* 1975-2010. Bethesda, MD: National Cancer Institute; 2013.

Time

Geller AC, Clapp RW, Sober AJ, et al. Melanoma epidemic: an analysis of six decades of data from the Connecticut Tumor Registry. *J Clin Oncol.* 2013;33:4172-4178.

Howlader N, et al. *SEER Cancer Statistics Review,* 1975-2010. Bethesda, MD: National Cancer Institute; 2013.

Migration and Disease Occurrence

Levine H, Afek A, Shamiss A, et al. Country of origin, age at migration, and risk of cutaneous melanoma: a migrant cohort study of 1,100,000 Israeli men. *Int J Cancer.* 2013;133:486-494.

Cohort Study

PATIENT PROFILE

A pediatrician was called to the hospital to attend the delivery of a newborn. The mother, a 28-year-old primigravida, had experienced elevated blood pressure during an otherwise uncomplicated pregnancy. The labor was induced because the pregnancy had continued 2 weeks past the expected date of fetal distress occurred. When the membranes ruptured, the obstetrician noted thick greenish fluid containing meconium was suctioned from his mouth and nose, the baby did not grimace, cough, or sneeze.

Vigorous efforts at resuscitation were initiated, including bag-and-mask ventilation with 100% oxygen and chest compressions, but the Apgar score at 1 minute of life was 1. The Apgar score (Table 5-1), an index of neonatal asphyxia, can range from 0 (very asphyxiated) to 10 (no asphyxia). Despite continuing resuscitation, the 5-minute Apgar score improved only to 2, with a heart rate of 110 beats/minute. The 10-minute Apgar score remained depressed at 3, and the neonate was transferred to Newborn Intensive Care Unit. With aggressive medical management, the 3100-g neonate continued to improve without evidence of acute neurologic com-plications. He was discharged from the hospital on the twelfth day of life.

CLINICAL BACKGROUND

Perinatal asphyxia can be defined as fetal hypoxia during labor and delivery. Hypoxia in the perinatal period is believed to be a major cause of both perinatal deaths and impaired development and neurologic function among survivors. The causes of perinatal asphyxia are not completely clear, but a number of factors have been associated with hypoxia during labor and delivery, including preeclampsia or eclampsia, maternal hypotension, placental insufficiency, and prematurity. The passage of meconium and presence of this material in the amniotic fluid indicate possible fetal distress.

The pathogenesis of perinatal asphyxia is presented in Figure 5-1. The development of severe metabolic acidosis in the fetus indicates a lack of oxygen. This is because tissues must resort to anaerobic glycolysis for energy production. The degree of hypoxia that a fetus can tolerate before cellular injury occurs is variable and depends on a variety of factors, including previous asphyxia during the pregnancy, metabolic needs versus metabolic reserves, and blood flow to vital organs.

Table 5-1 Apgar score for evaluation of neonatal asphyxia

Sign	score		
	0	1	2
Heart rate (beats/minute)	Absent	<100	>100
Respiration	Absent	Slow	Regular, crying
Muscle tone	Limp	Slow flexion	Active motor
Color	Blue, pale	Body pink, extremities blue	Completely pink
Reflex response to catheter in nostril	None	Grimace	Cough, sneeze

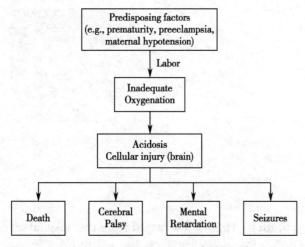

Figure 5-1. Schematic diagram of the pathogenesis of perinatal asphyxia.

In experimental studies on newborn primates, varying degrees of asphyxia have been induced. These studies have shown that for brain injury to occur, the fetus must be exposed to marked asphyxia for at least 25 minutes. These studies also indicate that this degree of asphyxia will probably lead to fetal death rather than survival with neurologic impairment. In general, research has shown that the immature nervous system is more resistant to hypoxia injury than the mature brain.

STUDY DESIGN

The parents of the newborn in the Patient Profile are understandably distraught by the unanticipated complications in their baby's first hours of life. Naturally, they have questions about what will bring in the future. Will their son develop normal mental capacity? Questions such as these from concerned parents often can be answered from the pediatrician's own clinical experience. Physicians who have seen only a few such patients, however, must consult the medical literature to respond to parental concerns.

In undertaking such a search, the pediatrician will find a variety of case reports concerning infants who have had severe perinatal asphyxia and have developed various acute and chronic medical problems. Some of these reports describe dismal outcomes, including death. However, there are also reports of instances of severe asphyxia during delivery in which the child later had normal neurologic development

and excellent school performance. Thus, the pediatrician may be uncertain about what to tell parents. Clearly, a broad spectrum of outcomes is possible. What the pediatrician in our case needs to find are studies that offer reliable evidence of the likelihood of each of the various possible outcomes.

The most definitive conclusions could be drawn from a clinical trial. This would be a study in which newborns are randomly assigned to groups with different levels of perinatal asphyxia and then followed with measurements of outcomes, such as achievement of developmental milestones and school performance on laboratory animals, but obviously such a study on human infants would be unethical. An investigator could not intentionally expose humans to potentially harmful conditions simply to learn about the effects on outcome.

Since intentional exposure of human newborns to asphyxia cannot be justified on ethical grounds, the investigator might resort to observing the outcomes of newborns who develop asphyxia under natural circumstances. This type of study is characterized as **observational study**, because the investigator does not determine the assignment of **exposure** but rather passively observes events as they unfold. The observational study design that is most similar to the clinical trial is a cohort study. In this type of study, as illustrated in Figure 5-2, the investigators identify a population (**cohort**) and determine their initial characteristics (exposure status). A cohort for an asphyxia study might consist of infants born with perinatal asphyxia and infants born without this condition. The researchers then follow the cohort over time and determine the outcome in the exposed and unexposed groups, it is important to remember that in a **cohort study,** information about the risk factor (exposure) is determined prior to the observation of disease status.

A large cohort study was conducted in the United States on the utility of Apgar scores as predictors of chronic neurologic disability. In this study, investigators evaluated 49,000 infants whose Apgar scores were recorded at 1 and 5 minutes of age. For those infants who did not achieve a score of 8 or higher at 5 minutes, Apgar scores were then recorded at 10, 15 and 20 minutes. All the children were then followed to the age of 7 years. The occurrence of seizures was determined through clinical observations in the newborn nursery; interval histories were recorded at 4, 8, 12, and 18 months of age and yearly thereafter. The presence of cerebral palsy was determined by physical examination at age 7 years. A psychological and developmental assessment was also performed at age 7. Then design of this study is shown in Figure 5-3.

This study demonstrated that low Apgar scores are risk factor for the development of cerebral palsy. However, 55% of the children with cerebral palsy at age 7 and Apgar scores of 7 or higher at 1 minute, and 73% scores 7 or higher at 5 minutes. Of the 99 children who survived and had Apgar scores of 0-3, at 10, 15, or 20 minutes, 12 were found to have cerebral palsy. Eleven of those 12 also had delayed metal development. Ten of those infants had seizures in the first 24 hours of life. Of the children who survived and had Apgar scores of 0-3 at 10 minutes or later, 80% were free of any major handicap at early school age.

This study of a large number of children provides the pediatrician in the Patient Profile with the kind of information needed to discuss the baby's prognosis with his parents. The study represents a range of experience that no individual practitioner could compile, even in a lifetime of practice. The pediatrician can now advise the parents that although their baby does have an increased risk of cerebral palsy and developmental delay, such an outcome occurs in only about one of eight asphyxiated neonates. Because the baby did not have a seizure in the first 24 hours of life, the prognosis may be more favorable. It should be reassuring to asphyxiated newborns were free of major neurologic handicap at early school age.

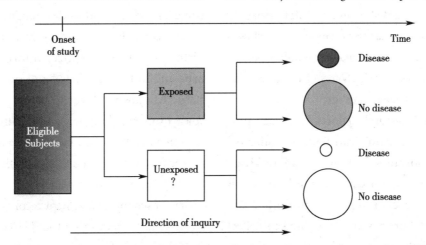

Figure 5-2. Schematic diagram of a cohort study. Shaded areas represent exposed population, and unshaded areas represent unexposed population.

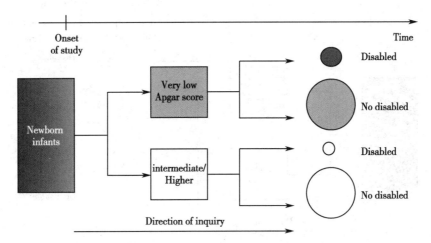

Figure 5-3. Schematic diagram of a cohort study of the relationship between perinatal asphyxia and chronic neurological disability. Shaded areas represent newborns with very low Apgar scores, and unshaded areas represent newborns with intermediate or high Apgar scores.

Perhaps the contributions of cohort studies can be illustrated best by the Framingham Heart Study, one of the most widely recognized and most influential studies of this type. In that investigation, the status of the residents of Framingham, Massachusetts, was determined with respect to potential risk factors for cardiovascular disease. Beginning in 1950, a sample of 6500 individuals aged 30-59 years was chosen form a total population of approximately 10,000 people in that age group. Approximately 5100 subjects with no clinical evidence of atherosclerotic cardiovascular disease agreed to participate in the study. Each subject was examined at the beginning of the study and was reexamined every 2 years thereafter. For example, the investigators identified subjects who had elevated blood pressure, subjects who smoked, and subjects who had elevated serum cholesterol levels. The population was followed over 35 years to identify subjects who suffered a myocardial infarction (MI), stroke, or other adverse cardiovascular event. This protocol allowed investigators to determine if an individual with hypertension, for example, was more likely to suffer a stroke than someone with normal blood pressure.

More than 250 research reports have been produced by the Framingham Heart Study investigators and their collaborators. The Framingham Heart Study is the source of our current knowledge about the risk factors for cardiovascular morbidity and mortality. This cohort has also been used to collect information regarding various other diseases.

Framingham was chosen as the site for the study for many reasons, but primarily because the community is stable and there is broad representation of occupations among the population. The Framingham study is limited, however, because its participants are mainly white, middle class individuals.

TIMING OF MEASUREMENTS

A cohort study is usually **prospective,** that is, exposure to the risk factor and subsequent health outcomes are observed after the beginning of the study (Figure 5-3). For example, a prospective cohort study of neonatal asphyxia and subsequent mental retardation could be started in 2000. The degree of neonatal asphyxia could be determined for births occurring though 2001, and the development of mental retardation could be assessed between 2001 and 2006, or later. An alternative name for such a cohort study is **longitudinal study**.

Occasionally, a cohort study is retrospective (or historic), that is, it utilizes information on prior exposure to the risk factor and subsequent disease status. As shown in Figure 5-4, a retrospective cohort study of neonatal asphyxia and neurologic disability designed in 2001 might involve a review of the medical records of infants born in a particular hospital in 1989 to determine the level of asphyxia, followed by a review of school achievement records over the period 1999-2000 to determine the degree of intellectual functioning. Note that exposure to risk factors and

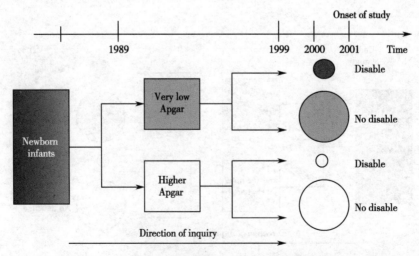

Figure 5-4. Schematic diagram of a retrospective cohort study of the relationship between perinatal asphyxia and chronic neurological disability. Shaded areas represent newborns with very low Apgar scores, and unshaded areas represent newborns with intermediate or high Apgar scores.

the subsequent development of the health outcome occur prior to the beginning of the retrospective.

The advantage of the retrospective cohort design is that all the events under study have already occurred, and conclusions can therefore be drawn more rapidly. In addition, the cost of a retrospective cohort study might be substantially lower for the same reason. The retrospective approach may also be the only feasible way to study the effects of an exposure that no longer occur, for example, discontinued medical treatments. On the other hand, a retrospective cohort study must usually rely on existing records or subject recall; both are usually less complete and accurate than data collected in a prospective study. Attributes of prospective and retrospective cohort studies are compared in Table 5-2.

Table 5-2 Comparison of the attributes of retrospective and prospective cohort studies

Attribute	Retrospective	Prospective Approach
Information	Less complete and accurate	More complete and accurate
Discontinues exposure	Useful	Not useful
Emerging new exposure	Not useful	Useful
Expense	Less costly	More costly
Completion	Shorter	Longer

It should now be clear that a prospective cohort study often takes a long time to complete. Furthermore, to ensure that there are enough subjects to reach a valid conclusion, a cohort study (either prospective or retrospective) usually requires a fairly large number of individuals with the potential to develop the outcome of interest. For example, in the study of perinatal asphyxia, data concerning 49,000 subjects were accumulated over a 7-year period. For this reason, such studies can be expensive to complete. In fact, if the outcome of interest under study is rare, the sample size required for a cohort study may be so large that it would be impractical to undertake such a study. On the other hand, if the exposure or risk factor is rare, a well-designed cohort study may offer superior statistical power to evaluate associations between exposure and subsequent development of disease, because this type of study allows selective inclusion of exposed persons. A cohort study of perinatal asphyxia, for example, could include all newborns with Apgar scores of 0-3 but only a sample of the large pool of newborns with higher scores.

Following subjects over a long period of time can lead to various problems. Subjects may move away or leave the study for other reasons, including death from cause other than the disease under investigation. If the losses to follow-up are substantial, and the lost subjects differ in outcome from those who remain in the study, the validity of the results can be affected seriously. It is also possible for exposure status to change during the course of the study. Obviously, birth asphyxia occurs only once. In other circumstances, however, the exposure under study may be subject to variation over time. For example, a cigarette smoker may quit, or, in an occupational cohort study, employees may change jobs and, therefore, their level of exposure to an occupational hazard may change. Diagnostic methods used for the disease under study may also vary over time.

The advantages and disadvantages of cohort studies are presented in Table 5-3.

Table 5-3 Advantages and disadvantages of cohort study

Advantages	Disadvantages
Direct calculation of risk ratio (relative risk)	Time consuming often requires a large sample size
May yield information on the incidence of disease	Expensive
Clear temporal relationship between exposure and disease	Not efficient for the study of rare diseases
Particularly efficient for study of rare exposures	Losses to follow-up may diminish validity
Can yield information on multiple exposures	Changes over time in diagnostic methods may lead to biased results
Can yield information on multiple outcomes of a particular exposure	
Minimizes bias	
Strongest observational design for establishing cause and effect relationship	

SELECTION OF SUBJECTS

Selection of subjects for a cohort study is influenced by various factors, including (1) the type of exposure under investigation, (2) the frequency of the exposure in the population, and (3) the accessibility of subjects and the likelihood of their continuing participation. Both exposed and unexposed groups must be free of the outcome of interest at the start of the study, and they must be similarly eligible to develop the outcome of interest during the course of the study. If some subjects already have the outcome of interest at the onset of the study, the temporal relationship between exposure and outcome will be obscured.

The Exposed Group

The type of exposure under investigation is critical for selection of the exposed group. Some exposures during pregnancy are common, such as gestational diabetes or hypertension. For these exposures, a general population of pregnant women could be used to construct the cohort. Other exposures, such as in vitro fertilization, are not common. In a cohort study designed to evaluate whether in vitro fertilization is a risk factor for developmental disability in the offspring, it may be necessary to sample exposed subjects from an infertility clinic rather than from among pregnant women in the general population.

Feasibility issues are also important in selecting the exposed population. The investigator should identify an accessible population that is motivated to participate in the study and unlikely to discontinue participation. The availability of historical information such as medical records may also be factor in selecting this group. Examples of groups that have been chosen for feasibility reasons include nurse, members of health maintenance organizations, residents of stable communities, and labor union members.

The degree of exposure may differ depending on the goals of the study. For some exposures, subjects are classified into one of two groups: exposed or unexposed. In vitro fertilization is an example of this type of dichotomization. Other studies involve a range of exposure levels, for example, Apgar scores as an indicator of perinatal asphyxia. The investigator may take a graded exposure variable, such as the Apgar score, and transform it into a categorical exposure by dividing subjects into those whose score exceeds a certain designated value (e.g., Apgar score of 3) and those whose score falls below that value. The value chosen to separate groups is referred to as a cutoff point and can be selected in various ways. For example, the cutoff point might be selected on the basic of the underlying distribution of value, such as the point that separates the 10% of subjects with the lowest Apgar scores from the remainder of the population. Alternately, a standard cutoff point can be used that is believed to have pathophysiologic implications, regardless of the underlying distribution in the population.

Thus, Apgar scores can be classified in the three different ways: dichotomous (0-3 versus >3), multiple ordered (0-3, 4-6, 7-10), or continuous (by gradation). If the exposure can be categorized into multiple levels or gradations, the investigator can determine whether a relationship exists between the dose (of the exposure) and the response. In the present context, the study may seek to determine whether the risk of chronic neurologic disability rises as the Apgar score decreases. If such a trend is observed, the argument that perinatal asphyxia is a cause of chronic neurologic disability is strengthened.

The Unexposed Group

Feasibility issues for the unexposed group are similar to those for the exposed group. The unexposed group must be accessible for entry into the study and for follow-up. When the purpose of a cohort study and is to investigate a community, such as in the Framingham Heart Study, that community is the source of the unexposed persons. Because there may be more unexposed people in the community than are needed for the investigation, a representative sample may be taken. In the Framingham Heart Study, several risk factors were of interest, all of which were relatively prevalent in the community. In this situation, a sample of the entire community was drawn and then subdivided into exposure groups, depending on the risk factor of interest in a particular analysis. In the study of perinatal asphyxia, the unexposed group was defined as the infants with the highest Apgar scores (7-10), indicating the lowest degree of perinatal asphyxia.

For cohort studies that involve the selection of a specific exposed population, selection of an appropriate comparison population may be less clear-cut. For example, in a study of in vitro fertilization as a risk factor for congenital malformations, the comparison group might be pregnant women who are followed in other obstetric practices. If, however, pregnant women in the comparison population are not followed with a comparable level of clinical scrutiny, or if the unexposed group of pregnant women differs from the exposed group of pregnant in other ways that might be related to congenital malformations, the study may lead to a false conclusion. The investigator may relate an observed increased risk of congenital malformation to in vitro fertilization when, in fact, the elevated risk is result of other differences between the exposed and unexposed groups. This type of problem illustrates why a randomized controlled clinical trial may be less susceptible to error than a cohort study. With randomization, factors known to be related to the development of disease—as well as other factors not yet recognized as related to the disease—tend to be balanced between the groups. This increases confidence that an observed association is, in fact, the result of the exposure of interest rather than the result of some other characteristic.

The underlying principle in selecting the unexposed group is that it should yield a fair comparison with the exposed group. Occasionally, the frequency of outcome occurs in the general population. This is particularly useful when members of the general population are very unlikely to be exposed to the study factor. However, the general population may not be comparable with those in the exposed group. For example, follow-up for disease occurrence may be more (or less) complete than for the exposed group. This may be lead to erroneous conclusions. Furthermore, if the exposed and unexposed are chosen from different time periods (a nonconcurrent study), medical care or other factors may differ between the groups in a way that makes the comparison unfair and the results invalid. Suggestions for the selection of exposed and unexposed are presented in Table 5-4.

DATA COLLECTION

The investigator must collect information on both the independent variable (exposure) and the dependent variable (response) during the course of a cohort study.

Exposure

It is essential to define the exposure clearly. Some exposures are acute, one-time episodes, never repeated in a subject's lifetime (eg, asphyxia at birth). Other exposures are long term, such as cigarette smoking or the use of oral contraceptives. Exposures

Table 5-4 Guidelines for selection of exposed and unexposed subjects in cohort studies.

Unexposed	Exposed	Unexposed and Exposed
Both exposed and unexposed groups should be free of the disease of interest and equally susceptible to development of the disease at the beginning of the study	The baseline characteristics of exposed persons should not differ systematically from those of unexposed persons, except for the exposure of interest	Unexposed persons should be sampled from the same (or comparable) source population as the exposed group
Equivalent information (quantity and quality) should be available on exposure and disease status in the exposed and unexposed groups		Multiple comparison groups of unexposed subjects chosen in different ways may reinforce the validity of findings
Both groups should be accessible and available for follow-up		

may also be intermittent, such as pregnancy-induced hypertension, which may occur during one pregnancy, disappear after delivery, and perhaps reappear during subsequent pregnancies. The types of exposure characteristics that should be considered are presented in Table 5-5.

Table 5-5 Measurements of exposure used in cohort studies

Measurements of Exposure	Example
Intensity	Mean blood pressure level
Duration	Weeks of hypertension
Regularity	Number of affected pregnancies
Variability	Range of measured blood pressure

A subject who originally satisfies the criteria for inclusion in a cohort study should not subsequently be excluded from the analysis because of a change in exposure status during follow-up. This type of exclusion may lead to biased conclusion. Specifically, it is possible that a change in exposure status may indicate a change in outcome status. For example, in a study of the relationship between the use of an antinausea medication during pregnancy and subsequent risk of spontaneous abortion, the medication may be discontinued for a subject because of early signs of threatened abortion. Excluding this subject from the analysis, therefore, may result in an underestimate of the true link between use of the medication and risk of abortion. The potential for changes in exposure status has important implications for the frequency of follow-up. Frequent reassessment of exposure and outcome status may be required if exposure status changes over time.

The source of available information about exposure may constrain the ability of the investigator to define and measure exposure experience. If the information comes from medical records, as is sometimes necessary in a retrospective cohort study, the accuracy of exposure information may be poor. For example, there are inherent disadvantages in using Apgar scores from medical records. Sometimes the Apgar scoring system is recorded by the medical staff as part of the required paperwork after delivery, without careful timing of the observations and detailed assessment by multiple observers. The medical staff providing patient care may be distracted by other responsibilities. In the previously cited prospective cohort study of neonatal asphyxia, a specially trained independent observer who was not responsible for patient care recorded the score in a standard manner on a standardized study form at exactly 1, 5, and 10 minutes of life.

In general, objective measures of exposure or biological markers of exposure are preferred over subjective measures. For example, in a study of maternal use of illicit drugs and pregnancy outcome, one approach to exposure assessment would be to question pregnant women about their use of illicit drugs. Self-reports of illicit drug use, however, are likely to under-represent actual exposure. Repeated measurements of drug metabolites in urine might provide a more accurate and reliable assessment of exposure.

Clinical response

Before, the start of the study, it is imperative to determine that subjects do not have the outcome (disease) under investigation. This may be particularly difficult if the outcome is a disease that develops slowly, has an insidious onset, and is asymptomatic until its late stages. One approach to this problem is to exclude cases in which the disease emerges early in the course of the investigation, under the assumption that the biological onset of disease preceded the beginning of the study.

The degree of surveillance for disease should be similar in the exposed and unexposed groups. The frequency of examination and the duration of follow-up depend on the type of exposure and the outcome under investigation. For some diseases, the time from exposure to development of disease is short. A cohort study of the relationship between exposure to perinatal asphyxia and death within the first week of life would have a short follow-up period. Other outcomes, such as chronic neurologic disability, may require years to assess. Because the investigators were interested in performance and cognitive ability at early school age, the study of the relationship of perinatal asphyxia to neurologic development required 7 years of follow-up.

Information on outcome status may come from various sources. Some cohort studies rely on information from the records of physicians and hospitals. This would be particularly pertinent for a cohort study focusing on a population with good access to health care and standardized recordkeeping practices, such as a prepaid health plan. Other cohort studies may combine physician records with periodic examinations by the investigators. The Framingham Heart Study is an example of this type of study. Another approach to collecting information on disease is to have the subjects report whether they develop the outcome of interest. The study may also involve reviews of medical records in a subset of subjects to confirm self-reports.

If the outcome under study is death from any cause, the investigator may use information from death certificates. Death certificates may have limited utility, however, if the study focuses on a specific disease, because cause-of-death information on death certificates may be inaccurate. Obviously, in that circumstance the best information would come from autopsy reports. This approach may not be feasible, however, since most people who die are not autopsies.

If diagnostic evaluations are required by the investigator during the study, an appropriate diagnostic test for the disease must be available (see chapter 8). This approach has limitations because diagnostic tests are not always available or feasible. To ensure a fair comparison between the exposed and unexposed groups, the accuracy and reliability of diagnosis must not differ between the groups. Thus, it can be helpful if those who assess outcomes are unaware of the subjects' exposure status. The study of perinatal asphyxia relied on standard neurologic examination and psychological tests. The examiners had no access to the medical records and, thus, were blind to the Apgar scores of the children. This blinded approach should facilitate an assessment of neurologic outcomes that is comparable for exposed and unexposed children.

It is possible for exposure status to alter the surveillance for disease. An example of this problem could occur in a study of neonatal asphyxia and intellectual development. Physicians are more likely to administer psychological and developmental tests to an infant who had a difficult birth with low Apgar scores; that child is, therefore, more likely to be diagnosed as having subtle developmental problems than another child who has not been singled out for close surveillance. This could lead to an overestimate of the relationship between neonatal asphyxia and subsequent developmental disability. This problem, however, can be avoided, as in the cited study, by ensuring that a standard diagnostic protocol is followed, regardless of exposure status.

ANALYSIS

Several different approaches can be used to analyze the results of a cohort study, as described in the following sections.

Risk Ratio

The results of a cohort study can be summarized using the format shown in Table 5-6. In that table, the letters *A-D* represent numbers of subjects in the four possible combinations of exposure and outcome status (in this instance, death).

Table 5-6 Summary of risk data from a cohort study

Outcome[a]	Exposed	Unexposed	Total
Death	A	B	A + B
No death	C	D	C + D
Total	A + C	B + D	A+B+C+D

[a] In some studies, the outcome is development of disease rather than death.

(A) Exposed persons who later die

(B) Unexposed persons who later die

(C) Exposed persons who do not die

(D) Unexposed persons who do not die

The total number of subjects in this study is the sum of A+B+C+D.

The total number of exposed persons is *A+C*, and the total number of unexposed persons is B+D.

Among exposed persons, the risk (R) of death is defined as

$$R_{(exposed)} = \frac{\text{Exposed persons who die}}{\text{All exposed persons}} = \frac{A}{A+C}$$

As indicated in Chapter 2, risk can vary between 0 (no exposed persons die) and 1 (all exposed persons die). As in all statements of risk, some time period for the development of the outcome must be specified. For example, the outcome might be the risk of death in the first year of life. Among unexposed persons, the risk of death is defined as

$$R_{(unexposed)} = \frac{\text{Unexposed persons who die}}{\text{All unexposed persons}} = \frac{B}{B+D}$$

One approach to contrasting the risk in two groups is to create a ratio measure. The **risk ratio** (RR) or relative risk is

$$RR = \frac{R_{(exposed)}}{R_{(unexposed)}} = \frac{A/(A+C)}{B/(B+D)}$$

If the exposed and unexposed persons have the same risk of death, the RR is 1 (e.g., the null value). That is, exposure is not related to the outcome. If the risk among exposed persons is greater than the corresponding risk among unexposed persons, the RR is greater than 1 (e.g., hazardous exposure). In contrast, if the risk among exposed persons is smaller than the corresponding risk among unexposed persons, the RR is less than 1 (e.g., beneficial exposure).

The calculation of risk ratio can be illustrated from the study of perinatal asphyxia. The data in Table 5-7 relate to infants who weighed more than 2500g at birth. Exposure is defined as an Apgar score of 0-3 at 10 minutes of life, and the comparison group of less exposed newborns had Apgar scores of 4-6 at 10 minutes. In the actual study, a third group with Apgar scores of 7-10 was included, but the data are not described here in detail.

The risk among exposed newborns is

$$R_{(exposed)} = \frac{42}{122} = 0.344 = 34.4\%$$

That is, about one of three newborns weighing more than 2500g and having very low Apgar scores at 10 minutes died during the first year of life. The risk among "less exposed" newborns is

$$R_{(unexposed)} = \frac{43}{345} = 0.125 = 12.5\%$$

Table 5-7 Relationship between 10-minute Apgar scores and risk of death in the first year of life among children with birth weights of at least 2500 g. [a]

	Apgar Score 0-3	Apgar Score 4-6	Total
Death	42	43	85
No death	80	302	382
Total	122	345	467

In other words, one in eight neonates weighing over 2500g and having intermediate Apgar scores at 10 minutes died during the first year of life.

Without any further calculations, it should be obvious that the neonates with very low 10-minute Apgar scores had a worse prognosis than those with intermediate 10-minute Apgar scores. Quantification of the magnitude of this effect is achieved by calculating the risk ratio

$$RR = \frac{R_{(exposed)}}{R_{(unexposed)}} = \frac{42/122}{43/345} = 2.8$$

The RR of 2.8 means that newborns at this birth weight with very low 10-minutes Apgar scores are almost three times more likely to die in the first year of life than similar-weighing newborns with intermediate 10-minute Apgar scores. The RR is a measure of the strength of association between exposure and outcome. The farther the RR is from the null value of 1, the stronger the association. The strength of association is an important criterion in evaluating whether an observed association is likely to represent a cause-and-effect relationship. The RR of 2.8 is consistent with a moderate-to-strong relationship between the exposure (10-minutes Apgar score) and outcome (infant death).

A sense of the statistical precision of this estimated risk ratio can be obtained by calculating **confidence intervals** around the point estimate of 2.8. The 95% confidence interval for the data presented in Table 5-7 is (1.9, 4.1). That is, at the 95% level of confidence, the range of RR values consistent with the observed data falls between 1.9 and 4.1. Thus, the data are consistent with a risk of death in infants with very low Apgar scores between roughly a doubling and a fourfold increase (Figure 5-5). The

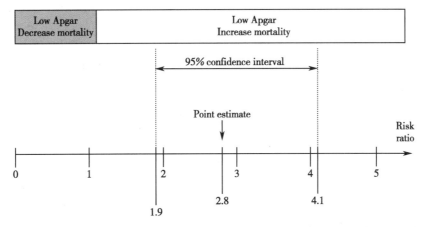

Figure 5-5. Point estimate and 95% confidence interval for risk ratio comparing infant mortality in newborns who weigh more than 2500g and have 10-minute Apgar scores of 0-3 with infant mortality for similar-weighing newborns with 10-minute Apgar scores of 4-6. (Data used, with permission, from Nelson KB, Ellenberg JH: Apgar scores as predictor of chronic neurologic disability. Pediatrics 1981;68:36.)

point estimate does not lie in the middle of the RR confidence interval. The asymmetry of this interval derives from the skew of the range of values of the risk ratio toward the positive direction (e.g., all beneficial effects are compressed into the range 0-1, whereas hazardous effects range from 1 to positive infinity).

Since the null value is excluded from this 95% confidence interval, it can be concluded that the findings are **statistically significant.** In other words, these data are not consistent with the null hypothesis of no association between Apgar scores and infant mortality (at the prespecified 95% level of confidence). An association as strong as that observed between Apgar scores and infant mortality, therefore, cannot be explained by chance alone.

As indicated earlier, the argument that the linkage between Apgar score and death in the first year of life is one of cause and effect is strengthened if a dose-response relationship can be demonstrated. A third group of newborns, with Apgar scores of 7-10, was therefore included in the study. Comparison of the risk of death in that group with the previous reference group, with had intermediate Apgar scores of 4-6, yields a risk ratio of 0.15, with an approximate 95% confidence interval of (0.11, 0.21). This result means that newborns with a 10-minute Apgar score of 7-10 have only about one-sixth the risk of death in the first year of life as newborns with Apgar scores of 4-6. This disparity is statistically significant, and

the very narrow width of the confidence interval indicates a statistically precise estimate (because it is based on a large number of observations).

The dose-response relationship between Apgar score and the risk ratio of death in the first year of life for newborns weighing more than 2500 g is shown in Figure 5-6. The reference group against which others were compared in the preceding calculations was the group with Apgar scores of 4-6 (e.g., the risk ratio for this group is defined as 1). A clear trend of decreasing risk ratio with increasing Apgar score is seen, and this trend is unlikely to have occurred by chance alone. Thus, there is strong evidence in these data for a dose-response relationship.

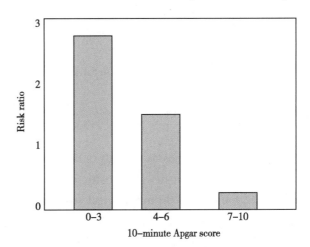

Figure 5-6. Dose-response relationship for the association between 10-minute Apgar scores and risk of death in the first year of life among newborns with a birth weight over 2500 g. (Data used, with permission, from Nelson KB, Ellenberg JH: Apgar scores as predictor of chronic neurologic disability. Pediatrics 1981;68:36.)

Attributable Risk

The risk of a specified outcome can be compared with measures other than a ratio. For example, the risk for one group can be subtracted from the risk for another group. This measure is termed the risk difference, or excess risk. Some authors use the term "attributable risk" for this measure, but that expression is discouraged here because it may be confused with other expression. The **risk difference** (RD) is defined as

$$RD = R_{(exposed)} - R_{(unexposed)} = \frac{A}{A+C} - \frac{B}{B+D}$$

Using the previously cited data relating 10-minute Apgar scores (0-3 versus 4-6) to the risk of death in the first year of life, we can calculate the risk difference as

$$RD = \frac{43}{122} - \frac{43}{345} = 0.344 - 0.125 = 0.129$$

That is, the risk of death in the first year of life is increased by 0.129 for newborns who weigh more than 2500 g and have a 10-minute Apgar score of 0-3, compared with similar-weighing newborns with a 10-minute Apgar score of 4-6.

Another measure of interest is the attributable risk percent (ARP), in which the risk difference is expressed as a percentage of the total risk experienced by the exposed group:

$$ARP = \frac{R_{(exposed)} - R_{(unexposed)}}{R_{(exposed)}} \times 100\%$$

$$= \frac{A/A+C - B/B+D}{A/A+C} \times 100\%$$

For the Apgar score-infant mortality data, the attributable risk percent is

$$ARP = \frac{0.344 - 0.125}{0.344} \times 100\% = 63.7\%$$

In other words, almost two thirds of the total risk of infant mortality for newborns who weigh more than 2500 g and have 10-minute Apgar scores of 0-3 is related to an Apgar score below the 4-6 level. The attributable risk percent typically is used as an indicator of the public health impact of exposure. These data suggest that birth asphyxia is a major contributor to—but not the sole cause of –infant mortality among severely asphyxiated children.

Rate Ratio

The analyses presented thus far are based on comparisons of risk estimates across exposure groups. In a cohort study, the measured outcome may be an incidence (or mortality) rate rather than a risk. Rate data in a cohort study can be summarized using the format shown in Table 5-8. The **rate ratio** is derived as follows

$$Rate\ ratio = \frac{Rate\ of\ outcome\ among\ exposed\ persons}{Rate\ of\ outcome\ among\ unexposed\ persons}$$

$$= \frac{A/PT_{(exposed)}}{B/PT_{(unexposed)}}$$

Table 5-8 Summary format of rate data from a cohort study

	Exposed Persons	Unexposed Persons	Total
Number of outcomes	A	B	A + B
Person-time (PT)	C	D	C + D

Table 5-9 Relationship between baseline serum cholesterol level and subsequent mortality rate from coronary heart disease among white males aged 25-39 at entry into the Chicago Heart Association Study[a]

	Cholesterol level		Total
	5.2-6.2 mmol/L[b]	≤5.1 mmol/L[c]	
Death	26	14	40
Person-years	36,581	68,239	104,820

[a] Data from Dyer AR, Stamler J, Shekelle RB: Serum cholesterol and mortality from coronary heart disease in young, middle aged, and other men and women from the three Chicago epidemiologic studies. Ann epidemiol 1992;2:51.

[b] 201-240 mg/dL

[c] ≤197 mg/ dL

The magnitude of the rate ratio is interpreted in the same manner as the risk ratio (<1= protective effect, 1= no effect, >1= harmful effect of exposure). The farther go away from the null value, the stronger association between exposure and the rate of the outcome will be showed. The data collected in the study of perinatal asphyxia were not presented in a manner that allows calculation of rate ratios.

To illustrate this measure, then, data are drawn from the Chicago Heart Association Detection Project in Industry (Dyer et al, 1992). That investigation involved almost 40,000 men and women at 84 cooperating companies and institutions in the Chicago area. Subjects were enrolled between 1967 and 1973, screened for risk factors for cardiovascular disease, and then followed an average 14-15 years. For white males aged 25-39 at entry, the relationship between baseline serum cholesterol levels and subsequent rate of coronary heart disease (CHD) is shown in Table 5-9. The rate ratio is

$$\text{Rate ratio} = \frac{26/36\,581}{14/68\,239} = 3.5$$

In other words, the mortality rate from CHD among white males with borderline high cholesterol levels was about 3.5 times higher than that of white males with lower cholesterol levels. Adjustment for underlying age differences in the study groups reduced the observed rate ratio to 3.1. Comparison of with high serum cholesterol levels (>6.2 mmol/L [>240mg/dL]) with white males of the same age with normal serum cholesterol levels (<5.1mmol/L [<197mg/dL]) yielded an age-adjusted rate ratio of 5.1. Thus, a dose-response relationship was evident between baseline serum cholesterol levels and subsequent CHD mortality.

SUMMARY

In this chapter, the basic approach to the design and analysis of cohort studies is presented, with illustrations drawn primarily from the literature on birth asphyxia. A **cohort study** is a type of observational investigation in which subjects are classified on the basis of level of exposure to a risk factor and followed to determine subsequent disease outcome. **Prospective cohort studies** are conducted by making all observations on exposure and disease status after the onset of the investigation. **Retrospective cohort studies** involve observations on exposure and disease status prior to the onset of the study. The retrospective approach offers several pragmatic advantages, but may result in less accurate and complete information on exposure and disease status.

Cohort studies are statistically efficient for the study of rare exposures because the exposed individuals can be selectively included in the study. On the other hand, cohort studies are inefficient for the investigation of slowly developing or rare diseases. The evaluation of chronic diseases through the cohort approach requires a long follow-up period and increases the chances that subjects will be lost from the study. The evaluation of rare diseases with the cohort study approach requires a large sample size and therefore is expensive and labor intensive. In order to improve research quality of cohort studies, and to evaluate the quality of published cohort studies, it is necessary to check if the method is appropriate or not. Therefore, the methodology checklist is recommended as the basis for judgment (Table 5-10).

There are several basic strategies to analyze cohort studies. If data are collected on the risk of developing an outcome during a specified period of time, the summary measure of effect typically is the risk ratio, or the risk of the outcome among exposed individuals. An alternative approach to contrasting risks is the **risk difference,** which is the risk among exposed persons minus the risk among unexposed persons. If the risk difference is divided by the risk among exposed persons, a measure termed the attributable risk percent is derived. The **attributable risk percent** is an indicator of the proportion of risk that may be attributable to the exposure per se. When data in a cohort study are based on the rate of disease outcome, the standard measure of effect is the **rate ratio.** Useful guide in evaluating the design and the analysis of published cohort studies.

The prospective cohort study of perinatal asphyxia cited in this chapter indicates that Apgar scores can serve a useful predictor of subsequent risk of death and neurologic disability. An inverse dose-response relationship occurs between Apgar score level and the risk of adverse neurologic outcome. In spite of the increased risk, however, most children with low Apgar scores survive and do not manifest neurologic or developmental disability. Through proper interpretation of the results of this cohort study, the pediatrician in the Patient Profile can inform the baby's parents that although their child faces an increased risk of certain disabilities, there is about an 80% chance that no neurologic handicaps will develop.

Table 5-10 Checklist for the evaluation of published cohort studies

Hypothesis

A. Is the study hypothesis clearly stated?

B. Does it address a question of clinical interest and important?

Design

A. Is the cohort design appropriate for the question to be answered?

B. Is it feasible to perform a cohort study?

Study Population

A. Will the study yield a fair comparison between the exposed and unexposed subjects?

B. Is the sample size adequate to answer the question of interest?

C. Are the exposed and unexposed subjects come from the same or different population?

D. Are the exposed and unexposed subjects examined concurrency?

E. Does the investigator present a rational for the choice of study population?

F. Is the study population similar to the type seen in clinical practice?

Exposure

A. Has the exposure been defined?

B. What is the source of exposure information?

C. Has the exposure been measured appropriately?

D. Are there objective measures or markers to substantiate subjective measures?

E. Is the exposure an acute or chronic one?

F. For chronic exposures, is there remeasurement during the course of the study?

G. Is it possible to examine a dose-response relationship?

Disease

A. Is the disease clearly defined?

B. What is the source of information about the disease?

C. Is there pathological or other confirmation of disease?

D. Has the presence of disease been assessed in a similar fashion for the exposed and unexposed groups?

E. Were those who assessed disease status blind to subject exposure status?

Follow-up

A. Was the period of follow-up adequate for the development of disease?

B. Were appropriate measures taken to maintain subjects in the study?

C. Is there discussion of losses to follow-up?

Analysis

A. Was an appropriate analysis performed?

B. Are the results statistically significant?

C. Are the results clinically meaningful?

(Zhibin Hu)

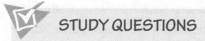

STUDY QUESTIONS

Directions: *For each question, select the single best answer.*

Questions 1-5: A cohort study is conducted to evaluate the relationship between dietary fat intake and the development of prostate cancer in men. In the study, 100 men with a high fat diet are compared with 100 men who are low fat diet. Both groups start at age 65 and are followed for 10 years. During the follow-up period, 10 men in the high fat intake group are diagnosed with prostate cancer and 5 men in the low fat intake group develop prostate cancer.

1. *What is the risk of the developing prostate cancer in the high fat group?*

   A. *0.05* B. *0.10*

   C. *0.15* D. *0.20*

   E. *0.25*

2. *What is the risk of the developing prostate cancer in the low fat group?*

   A. *0.05* B. *0.10*

   C. *0.15* D. *0.20*

   E. *0.25*

3. *What is the risk ratio (high fat consumers compared to low fat consumers) for the occurrence of prostate cancer?*

   A. *0.05* B. *0.75*

   C. *1.0* D. *1.5*

   E. *2.0*

4. *The point estimate for the risk ratio in question 3 suggests that the risk of prostate cancer associated with consumption of a high fat diet is*

   A. *decreased.*

   B. *increased.*

   C. *not affected.*

   D. *cannot be determined from the information provided.*

5. *The 95% confidence interval is 0.95 to 3.5. For statistical significance at an alpha level of 0.05, the correct interpretation of these results is that*

   A. *A statistically significant association exists between high dietary fat intake and an increased risk for prostate cancer.*

B. *A statistically significant association exists between high dietary fat intake and an decreased risk for prostate cancer.*

C. *It can be concluded with 95% CI that high dietary fat intake protects against prostate cancer.*

D. *It can be concluded with 95% CI that high dietary fat intake increase the risk of prostate cancer.*

E. *The risk of prostate cancer is not statistically significantly different between men with high fat intake and men with low fat intake.*

Question 6-10: A cohort study is conducted to evaluate the relationship between serum cholesterol level and the occurrence of myocardial infarction in women. In the study, 500 women with high serum cholesterol levels and 500 women without high serum cholesterol levels are followed over a 10-year period. During the study, 40 of the women with high serum cholesterol levels and 15 of the women with normal serum cholesterol levels develop a newly diagnosed myocardial infarction.

6. *The incidence rate (per 10,000 person-years) for a myocardial infarction among women with high serum cholesterol is*

   A. *30.*   B. *50.*

   C. *60.*   D. *80.*

   E. *100.*

7. *The incidence rate (per 10,000 person-years) for a myocardial infarction among women with normal serum cholesterol is*

   A. *30.*   B. *50.*

   C. *60.*   D. *80.*

   E. *100.*

8. *The (incidence) rate ratio for myocardial infarction is*

   A. *0.37.*   B. *1.33.*

   C. *2.67.*   D. *3.15.*

   E. *3.75.*

9. *The risk difference is*

   A. *0.002.*   B. *0.005.*

   C. *0.006.*   D. *0.01.*

E. *0.05.*

10. *the attributable risk percent is*

   A. *25.5%.*   B. *35.0%.*

   C. *47.5%.*   D. *55.5%.*

   E. *62.5%.*

IMPORTANT TERMINOLOGY

cohort study	队列研究
retrospective cohort study	历史性队列研究
prospective cohort study	前瞻性队列研究
longitudinal study	纵向研究
exposure	暴露
risk ratio	危险比
rate ratio	率比
attributable risk	归因危险度
risk difference	率差

FURTHER READING

Rothman KJ, Greenland S,Lash T L. Modern epidemiology. 3rd Edition. Lippincott Williams & Wilkins. 2008.

W. Ahrens, I. Pigeot. Handbook of Epidemiology. Bremen Institute for Prevention Research and Social Medicine (BIPS). Berlin, Germany. 2006; 474-477.

Goldberg RJ, McManus DD, Allison J. Greater knowledge and appreciation of commonly used research study designs. Am J Med. 2013;126:169e1-e8.

Thiese MS. Observational and interventional study design types; an overview. Biochmia Medica. 2014;24:199-210.

REFERENCES

Porta M. A dictionary of epidemiology. 5th.edition. New York: Oxford University Press, 2008. ISBN 978-0-19-531450-2 and ISBN 0-19-531450-6 [1] (the 6th. was published in June 2014)

Raymond Greenberg. Medical Epidemiology: Population Health and Effective Health Care. 5th edition.McGraw-Hill Education (LANGE Basic Science)

Case-Control Study

HEALTH SCENARIO AND CLINICAL BACKGROUND

In 1995, Early Breast Cancer Trialists' Collaborative Group compared treatments for early breast cancer. It showed that hormonal and cytotoxic therapies definitely improved 10-year survival, but radiotherapy did not, perhaps because moderate protection was counterbalanced by a moderate increase in risk. Although radiotherapy plus surgery was associated with a reduced risk of death due to breast cancer, but there were no definite differences in overall survival at 10 years compared to surgery alone. Nearly breast cancer, surgery can remove any disease that has been detected in or around the breast or regional lymph nodes, but undetected deposits of disease may remain either locally (i.e., in the residual breast tissue, scar area, chest wall, or regional lymph nodes) or at distant sites that could, if untreated, develop into life-threatening recurrence. National Institutes of Health (NIH) recommended that after breast-conserving surgery (BCS) there should be radiotherapy to the conserved breast. Breast radiotherapy immediately after BCS could improve long-term survival (by comparison with a policy of watchful waiting for any local recurrence) only if life-threatening spread from tumor cells in the conserved breast would otherwise occur after BCS but before any clinically evident local recurrence was detected and treated, or if the local disease could then not be controlled adequately. Hence, radiotherapy is likely to have little effect on early mortality, whatever effect it might have on long-term breast cancer mortality, that radiotherapy for early-stage breast cancer can reduce the rate of recurrence and of death from breast cancer.

However, long-term follow-up in some trials has shown that radiotherapy can increase the risk of ischemic heart disease, presumably through incidental irradiation of the heart. Radiotherapy regimens for breast cancer have changed since the women in these trials were irradiated, and the doses of radiation to which the heart is exposed are now generally lower. Nevertheless, in most women, the heart still receives doses of 1 to 5 Gy. Several studies have suggested that exposures at this level can cause ischemic heart disease, but the magnitude of the risk after any given dose to the heart is uncertain, as are the time to the development of any radiation-related disease and the influence of other cardiac risk factors. In 2013, Darby et al conducted a study relating the risk of ischemic heart disease after radiotherapy to each woman's radiation dose to the heart and to any cardiac risk factors she had at the time of radiotherapy. In this chapter, we will explore how the radiotherapy association with ischemic heart disease can be explored using the case-control research approach.

INTRODUCTION

Chapter 5 discussed that the basic design of a **cohort study** is to **sample** subjects based on their being exposed or not and then to follow them for subsequent development of the outcome. A **sample** starts with an outcome then traces back to investigate exposure. Instead of sampling exposed and unexposed persons, the investigator of a case-control study samples persons with the outcome of interest (cases) and constructs a comparison group (controls) of individuals who do not have the outcome of interest. Porta's Dictionary of Epidemiology defines the case-control study as: an **observational epidemiological study** of persons with the disease (or another outcome variable) of interest and a suitable control group of persons without the disease (comparison group, reference group). The potential relationship of a suspected risk factor or an attribute to the disease is examined by comparing the diseased and non-diseased subjects with regard to how frequently the factor or attribute is present (or, if quantitative, the levels of the attribute) in each of the groups (diseased and non-diseased). The design of the case-control study is illustrated in Figure 6-1. In essence, the study starts on the right hand side of the diagram with the identification of cases and controls. It then "looks backward in time" to identify earlier exposure patterns among the subjects. If it turns out that more cases than controls had an exposure of interest, it may be evidence that exposure is associated positively with outcome (i.e., exposure increases the risk of disease development). However, if cases are less likely than controls to have had the exposure of interest, it may constitute evidence that exposure is associated inversely with outcome (e.g., exposure decreases the risk of disease development).

The major difference between cohort and case-control methods is in the selection of the study subjects. In a cohort study, we start by selecting subjects who are initially free of disease and classify them according to their exposure to putative risk factors, whereas in a case-control study, we identify subjects on the basis of presence or absence of the disease (or any other outcome) under study and determine past exposure to putative risk factors. In many situations, however, a case-control study is more efficient than a cohort study because a smaller sample size is required. In a well-designed case-control study, cases are selected from a clearly defined population, sometimes called the **source population**, and controls are selected from the same population that yielded the cases. In order for the case-control study to estimate the association between the exposure and disease of interest, the exposure distribution among the population which produced these cases needs to be known.

The approach to the design of a case-control study can be illustrated by one study, conducted in Sweden and Denmark (Darby et al, 2013), designed to assess the association between radiation dose at the time of radiotherapy for breast cancer and the risk of ischemic heart disease. In this study, investigators identify all cases of ischemic heart disease occurred after a diagnosis of breast cancer but before any recurrence or diagnosis of a second cancer. They selected control at random from all eligible women in the study population. Patient records from hospital oncology departments were used to obtain data on each woman's medical history before her diagnosis of breast cancer, tumor characteristics, and radiotherapy. A total of 963 women with major coronary events and 1205 controls were included in the study.

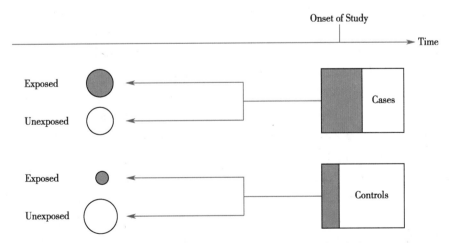

Figure 6-1. Illustration of the design of a case-control study. Shaded areas represent exposed persons, and unshaded areas represent unexposed persons.

Women irradiated for cancer of the left breast had higher rates of major coronary events than women irradiated for cancer of the right breast. The risk of a major coronary event increased linearly with the mean dose to the heart. Rates of major coronary events increased linearly with the mean dose to the heart by 7.4% per gray (95% confidence interval, 2.9 to 14.5), with no apparent threshold. The increase started within the first 5 years after radiotherapy and continued into the third decade after radiotherapy.

Case-control study illustrates several important features. First, the design provides an efficient means to study rare diseases. Case-control studies tend to be more feasible than other types of epidemiologic investigations, such as cohort studies, because fewer subjects are required. The smaller sample size is accompanied by a reduction in cost. Second, case-control studies allow researchers to investigate several **risk factors.** In this example, the investigators evaluated radiotherapy and other factors as possible causes of ischemic heart disease. Third, as with other non-experimental or observational studies, a single case-control investigation does not "prove" causality, but it can provide suggestive evidence of a causal relationship that warrants intervention by public health officials to reduce exposure to the implicated risk factor.

CASE

A case in a case-control study is an individual who is diagnosed with a disease of interest or a particular condition under investigation. A clear and valid case definition is important for any type of case-control study, and is especially important for case-control studies because the case definition will be used to define the study population, from which control subjects will be selected.

It is important to establishing the definition of a case is to identify the sampling frame from which cases will be selected. At least two different general approaches warrant further discussion. One is to choose a **hospital-based** sample, which generally means finding the cases from medical records in hos-

pitals and outpatient clinics, laboratories and other diagnostic facilities, reimbursement data, and other registration systems. The advantages of this approach are that it is efficient, cost effective, and fast. It can also simplify the selection of controls if they are sampled from other patients (e.g.,without ischemic heart disease) who are treated at those same facilities.

The counterpart to a hospital-based case-control study is a **population-based** case-control study. Here, the intent is to identify all of the cases that arise within a population. Typically, the population is defined by place of residence, such as within a particular city, region, or state. The population could be defined by other parameters, however. For example, one could select the population of interest on the basis of occupation or participation in a particular health insurance plan. A population-based study has the advantage of potentially more complete case finding and avoiding potential pitfalls of referral patterns. Because controls can be selected from the same well-defined source population, they may constitute a more representative and unbiased comparison group. The challenges of a population-based study are pragmatic concerns, such as potentially greater time and expense to complete.

CONTROLS

In a case-control study, controls are the persons who do not have the disease of interest or condition under investigation. Although the selection of cases may seem to be the complicated sampling issue in a case-control study, it turns out that there are at least as many considerations in the selection of controls. The guiding principle for control selection is that they should come from the same population as gave rise to the cases. Another way of expressing this concept is to choose controls who would have been included as cases, had they developed the disease of interest.

The sources for control selection are finalised once the study investigators agree on the target study population. The control selection must follow the population definition, because the controls are representative sample of the population which produced the cases. If the study is a population-based case-control study, the controls must be selected from the clearly specified population; that is, from those who satisfy the population definition, but without the disease of interest at the time when the disease in the cases was diagnosed. If the case group consists of all the cases produced by the specified population during the study period, then the best control group would be a **random sample** from those who have not developed the disease of interest at the time of the control selection. For example, the previously mentioned population-based case-control study of exposed to ionizing radiation during radiotherapy for breast cancer and the risk of ischemic heart disease ascertained and recruited the cases from Sweden and Denmark during the study period. The study selected its population-based controls at random from all eligible women by frequency-matching the cases on the basis of country of residence, age at the time of breast-cancer diagnosis, and year of diagnosis, with both age and year matched within 5 years for control.

For hospital-based studies, if the study is conducted in a hospital or clinic, the investigators must first define the members of the population which produced these hospitalized patients. The controls can be selected from the persons who seek medical services at the same hospitals as the cases, or from the patients seeking medical care at other hospitals which usually refer patients to the study hospitals. For example, a case-control study was conducted to explore a causal association between human papillomavirus (HPV) and oropharyngeal cancers. The control group consisted of patients without a history of cancer who were seen for benign conditions in the same clinic from which the case patients were enrolled. Subsequent to enrollment of a case, eligible control patients within the same sex and 5-year age categories were approached until two control patients were individually matched to each case patient. This tends to reduce or eliminate any distortion that might arise from selective referral patterns to the facilities of interest. One often used guideline is to sample controls from patients admitted with a number of different diagnoses so that the controls are not unduly weighted by a risk factor profile of one or a few conditions. Another frequent guideline is to sample controls preferentially from patients with acute diagnoses so that they do not have a long-standing condition that could distort their exposure history.

MATCHING

Matching is usually used in control selection when major confounders need to be controlled. In case-control studies, matching means requiring the controls to have the same or similar distribution for the matched variables as the cases. So, for example, we might choose for a white, female case who is age 65 years a white, female control of similar age(±5 years). We refer to this person-to-person alignment of cases and controls as matching. Another way of expressing this process is that controls are selected to parallel selected attributes of cases, such as demographic characteristics.

The motivation for matching usually is to remove any disparity in these characteristics between the groups under comparison. There are two reasons for wanting to remove the influences of these other variables. The first is to promote the study efficiency. This is because matching in a case-control study ensures an adequate number of cases and controls for each level or each combination of the matched factors and, therefore, matching permits effective control of **confounding** from the matched factors in data analysis. Otherwise, there may be only cases or controls if the study totally relies on stratification to control confounding from the matched confounders. A second motivation for matching is to to reduce the potential for confounding. Confounding may be present when the persons who have the exposure of interest also have other risk factors that are less common in unexposed persons.

The study can select either **frequency matching (or group matching)** or individual matching in selecting the controls in order to achieve this end. Population-based case-control studies usually use frequency matching, which requires the frequency distribution of the matching variables in the controls to be identical to that of the case group if the matched variable is a **categorical variable** (such as gender) or similar to the case group if the matched variable is a **continuous variable** (such as age). For instance, if 25% of the cases are males aged 65-75 years, 25% of the controls would be taken to have similar characteristics. Frequency matching within rather broad categories is sufficient in most studies. **Individual matching** can be performed on a one case-to one control basis (pair matching). Alternatively, one often sees two, three, or more controls matched for each case. Enlarging the number of controls per case increases the statistical power of the study. This maybe an important consideration for rare diseases where the number of eligible cases is limited. However, one reaches the point of diminishing returns in terms of statistical power by increasing the size of the control group. Typically, there is minimal gain in precision beyond a ratio of four controls per case. In the instance of the cited study of radiotherapy and ischemic heart disease, for example, the matching ratio was one control for per case in Sweden and two controls for per case in Denmark. The number of characteristics for which matching is desirable and practical is actually rather small. It is usually sensible to match cases and controls only for characteristics such as age, sex and ethnicity whose association with the disease under study is well known.

If matching is performed, a slightly different tabular summary (see in analysis section) and analysis must be performed taking into account the matching in the design. The results of a matched and an unmatched analysis may give similar results, but this is not guaranteed, and the preferred approach on both validity and precision grounds is to consider the matching in the analysis.

EXPOSURE

After the cases and controls have been selected, the next task is to collect information on the **exposure** of interest. Based on the specific hypothesis and aims, a case-control study must decide: (1)What information will be collected? (2) What are the sources for the information? And, (3) How will the information be collected? Because the exposures all occurred in the past, there may be real constraints in terms of the sources of information, as well as the level of completeness and accuracy. In a case-control study, it is a challenge to collect information on a wide range of exposures without affecting study efficiency. A variety of methods may be considered for collecting exposure information.

One of the most common strategies is to conduct direct interviews with cases and controls or ask them to complete questionnaires. And structured questionnaire is the most frequently used technique to obtain exposure information in case-control studies. To ensure that information from cases and controls is obtained in the same manner, interviews should be standardized, monitored, and conducted by trained interviewers. Interviews and questionnaires generally involve minimal burden on the subjects and can be completed relatively quickly and inexpensively. At the same time, interview data are imperfect at best because the ability of subjects to recall exposures can be highly variable, especially for exposures that occurred many years earlier. In addition, often there is concern that the recall of earlier events will differ systematically between cases and controls. Specifically, people may be more likely to search for explanation for the disease in the cases and, therefore, may assign more significance to past events. Controls, especially if they are healthy or have only an acute illness, have a different mindset and may not be as thorough in their recall. It is also possible that cases may tend to over report actual exposures, especially if they have done research on their illnesses and are aware of suspected risk factors, including the focus of the study. Whether the source of the **bias** is over reporting of true exposures in cases or underreporting of true exposures in controls, the net effect of the situation is to exaggerate the magnitude of the difference between cases and controls in reported rates of exposure to risk factors under investigation. To the extent possible, one would like to blind the interviewers and respondents to the exposure of interest and to ask about a variety of exposures so that the exposure of interest is not obvious. Whenever possible, it also is beneficial to validate reported exposure histories through other data sources. It is also desirable to assess the reliability of the questionnaire or interview by asking a sample of subjects the same questions at different points in time and looking for consistency across the responses.

Another common approach to collecting information on exposure is to access medical, education, work, or other record sources. This is particularly relevant for a study of radiotherapy for breast cancer because individual patient information and individual radiotherapy charts, including a diagram or photograph of the treatment fields and a dose plan were obtained from hospital records. This information tends to be fairly accurate and complete. For each woman, the mean radiation doses to the whole heart and to the anterior descending coronary artery were estimated from her radiotherapy chart. However, the problem is that most of the historical records collected are not for scientific purposes, and their completeness and accuracy on the exposure of interest is usually questionable. The level of missing or incomplete information can be substantial. Statistical methods can be used to impute missing values, but this is sophisticated guesswork and has uncertainty associated with it. Inaccurate information, whether from records or recall, if it arises similarly for cases and controls, will serve to make it more difficult to detect a true exposure-disease association. That is, any bias will be a conservative one. If an association is still observed despite the misclassified exposure information, the true association is expected to be as large as or larger than the magnitude observed.

A third approach to collecting information on exposure is to have some direct or indirect measurement of it. For example, one might be able to measure blood levels of certain agents. This is particularly helpful if there are appropriately stored specimens (e.g., umbilical cord blood) that can be assessed for cases and controls. And the specimens would have to be stored without degradation or compromise for many years or decades. Epidemiological studies are more and more reliant on laboratory-based measurements of environment or **biomarkers** to study exposure-disease relationship because these exposure assessments can directly assess body burden, internal dose, biologically active dose, or susceptibility biomarkers. Laboratory-based measurements of environment exposures or exposure biomarkers can be very valuable if historically collected environmental or biological samples are available, and the measured exposure represents the actual exposure associated with disease development.

ANALYSIS

In the most basic form of analysis, for a case-control study, both disease status (case vs. control) and exposure status (exposed vs. unexposed) are treated as simple dichotomous variables. In such a situation, there are four possible classifications of individual subjects:

a. Cases who were exposed

b. Controls who were exposed

c. Cases who were not exposed

d. Controls who were not exposed

We can summarize these four groups in a tabular format as illustrated in Table 6-1. This display appears identical to the 2×2 table introduced in the analysis of cohort studies (See Chapter 5).

Table 6-1 Summary format for data collected in a case-control study

	Case	Control	Total
Exposed	a	b	a+b
Unexposed	c	d	c+d
Total	a + c	b + d	a + b + c + d=n

For discontinuous variable, the chi-square test is the simplest method to determine whether observed differences in proportion between study groups. The chi-square statistic for a two-by-two table can be expressed as follows:

$$\chi^2 = \frac{(ad-bc)^2 n}{(a+b)(c+d)(a+c)(b+d)}$$

Nevertheless, the approach to sampling in cohort studies (based on exposure status) is fundamentally different from that in case-control studies (based on disease status). In a case-control study, the investigator determines the ratio of cases (a+c) to controls (b+d) and thereby sets the proportion of individuals in the study who are affected by the disease.

We begin by considering the exposure probability among cases, or the proportion of cases who were exposed previously. Using the notation introduced in **Table 6-1**, we calculate this probability as:

$$\text{case exposure probability} = \frac{\text{Exposed cases}}{\text{All cases}} = \frac{a}{a+c}$$

The odds of a case being exposed are estimated by the probability of a case being exposed divided by the probability of a case being unexposed. This measure is calculated as:

$$\text{Odds of case exposure} = \frac{\dfrac{\text{Exposed cases}}{\text{All cases}}}{\dfrac{\text{Unexposed cases}}{\text{All cases}}}$$

$$= \frac{a}{a+c} \bigg/ \frac{c}{a+c} = \frac{a}{c}$$

Using a comparable calculation, the odds of exposure among controls can be shown to be estimated by:

$$\text{Odds of control exposure} = \frac{b}{d}$$

The ratio of these two odds (odds of exposure among cases divided by odds of exposure among controls) is referred to as the **odds ratio** (OR). The OR is calculated as:

$$OR = \frac{\text{Odds of case exposure}}{\text{Odds of control exposure}} = \frac{\dfrac{a}{c}}{\dfrac{b}{d}} = \frac{a \times d}{b \times c}$$

The exposure odds ratio is usually used to the risk in a case-control study. An exposure odds ratio mathematically equals a risk odds ratio if the data from the case-control study is valid. And, if the disease is rare, a risk odds ratio can be used to estimate the risk ratio. That is the very reason why, while the goal of an aetiological study is to find out the probability of developing disease among the exposed and non-exposed people, we can still use exposure odds ratio to estimate the magnitude of the association between the exposure and the disease of interest, although the case-control study signifies the probability of exposure among the cases and the controls.

When newly diagnosed (incident) cases are sampled from the same source population as controls, and sampling is independent of exposure history (all features of a well-designed case-control study), it can be shown that the OR gives an approximation to the incidence rate ratio. So, although the OR is a distinct measure of association and the preferred measure in a case-control study, it has an interpretation analogous to the rate ratio or risk ratio. The null value (no association) of the OR is 1.0. Values of the OR greater than 1.0 indicate a positive association between exposure and disease. Values of the OR below 1.0 indicate an inverse association between exposure and disease. It is important to calculate a **confidence interval** for each odds ratio. A confidence interval that includes 1.0 means that the association between the exposure and outcome could have been found by chance alone and that the association is not statistically significant. An odds ratio without a confidence interval is not very meaningful.

The formula for the confidence interval can be expressed as follows:

$$\ln OR 95\% CI = \ln OR \pm 1.96\sqrt{Var(LnOR)}$$

To illustrate the calculation of an OR, let us consider a case-control study of HPV exposure and oropharyngeal cancer conducted by D'Souza and colleges (2007). The investigators identified newly diagnosed patients in the outpatient otolaryngology clinic. The control group consisted of patients without a history of cancer who were seen for benign conditions in the same clinic from which the case patients were enrolled. Two controls were individually matched to each case patient. Specimens were collected from case patients before therapy and control patients at enrollment, and were used to detect of HPV. A summary of the data that were observed is shown in **Table 6-2**.

Table 6-2 Summary of data on the association of oral HPV infection with oropharyngeal cancer

Oral HPV-16 infection	Case	Control	Total
Positive	32	8	40
Negative	68	192	260
Total	100	200	300

Data from Gypsyamber D'Souza, Aimee R. Kreimer, Raphael Viscidi, Michael Pawlita, Carole Fakhry, Wayne M. Koch, William H. Westra, and Maura L. Gillison. Case–Control Study of Human Papillomavirus and Oropharyngeal Cancer. *The new England Journal of medicine.* 2007; 356; 1944-56

$$\chi^2 = \frac{(ad-bc)^2 n}{(a+b)(c+d)(a+c)(b+d)}$$

$$= \frac{(32\times192 - 8\times68)^2 \times 300}{40\times260\times100\times200} = 45.2$$

So because $P<0.01$, the result showed statistical significance and revealed that HPV exposure is associated with oropharyngeal cancer.

The OR calculated from these data would be:

$$OR = \frac{a\times d}{b\times c} = \frac{32\times192}{8\times68} = 11.3$$

In other words, the oral HPV-16 infection subjects are 11.3 times as likely to develop the oropharyngeal cancer as the non-infected. As with risk ratios, 95% confidence intervals (CIs) can be calculated around the point estimate of the OR. The approximate 95% CI for this OR is (5.0, 25.7). Because it excludes the null value (OR =1.0), we can conclude that the observed association is unlikely to have arisen from chance alone. Thus, if an odds ratio (OR), for example, has a 95% CI that excludes 1.0 and is relatively narrow, then we can be more confident in concluding that the observed association is unlikely to be due to random error or chance. The strength of the association, as judged by the distance from the null value, nevertheless, may be characterized as relatively weak. As a rough guideline for interpretation, a moderate association would correspond to an OR approaching 2, and a relatively strong association would correspond to an OR of 3 or greater. These are somewhat subjective interpretations; however, a relatively weak strength of association may still have public health importance if the exposure is common and the disease involves appreciable morbidity and mortality.

In a matched case-control study, the analysis must account for the matched sampling scheme. When one control is matched to each case, summary data can be presented in the format shown in **Table 6-3**. An extension of this basic format can be employed for situations in which the ratio of controls to cases differs from 1:1. Although there are four cells in **Table 6-3**, the entries into this format are quite different from what we find in previous tables (**Table 6-1**). Each entry into **Table 6-3** represents not one subject but two (a matched case-control pair). That is, each case-control pair can be classified into one of the four basic combinations of exposure status:

Table 6-3 Layout of a 2×2 table with data from an individual-matched case–control study (control-to-case ratio = 1:1)

	Case		
Control	**Exposed**	**Unexposed**	**Total**
Exposed	a	b	a+b
Unexposed	c	d	c+d
Total	a+c	b+d	a+b+c+d

In the table, a, b, c, d represent the number of pairs in which

a. Both case and control exposed (++)

b. Case unexposed but control exposed (+−)

c. Case exposed but control unexposed (−+)

d. Both case and control unexposed(−−)

Case-control pairs that are entered into cells a and d are referred to as concordant pairs, because, in these pairs, the exposure status of cases and controls is the same. Case-control pairs that are entered into cells b and c, in contrast, are referred to as discordant pairs because, in these pairs, the exposure status of cases and controls differs. It can be explained intuitively: pairs where both case and control were exposed or where both were unexposed give no information about the relationship of the exposure to disease.

The first step is to determine whether observed differences in proportions between study groups are statistically significant with the chi-square test as follows:

$$\chi^2 = \frac{(b-c)^2}{(b+c)}$$

When b + c<40, the adjusted formula:

$$\chi^2 = \frac{(|b-c|-1)^2}{b+c}$$

The OR for a 1:1 pair-matched case-control study is given by a simple ratio:

$$OR = \frac{c}{b}$$

This odds ratio can be interpreted in the same manner as the OR for unmatched studies. The calculation of OR 95% CI can use different methods, including the one shown above described by Woolf.

SUMMARY

In this chapter, we introduced another important type of observational research design referred to as a case-control study. This type of research approach is particularly well suited to the study of rare diseases and those with long developmental (latent) periods. The case-control study begins with the sampling of cases (persons with the disease of interest). A comparison group (controls) without the disease of interest then is selected. And controls are a representative sample of the population which produced these cases.

■ **Cases** often are sampled from one or more hospital or other clinical facilities (a hospital-based sample). Identification of cases can be made from the general population using health register (population-based sample) and data or from a particular medical setting. Information on diseases can be got from death certificates, disease registers, medical records or population survey. For rare diseases, cases may have to seek from large areas or over many years. Population based case control studies are generally more expensive and difficult to conduct.

■ Define and select controls are very important steps. **Controls** should be chosen who are similar in many ways to the cases, except they do not have the outcome of interest. The factors (e.g., age, sex, time of hospitalisation) chosen to define how controls are to be similar to the cases are the 'matching criteria'. In order to minimize bias, controls should be selected to be a representative sample of the population which produced the cases.

■ **Matching** of cases and controls can eliminate the matched parameter as a cause of difference. Controls are matched to cases on the basis of certain characteristics, which are also known to be present in the cases. The purpose is to eliminate confounding variables (described in Chapter 9). If such confounding factors are unevenly distributed between study groups, they can distort comparisons and the conclusions being made. Matching should be used sparingly. The tendency is to match in analysis of results rather than in the design stage. Overmatching occurs if a variable matched could, in fact be an intermediate on a casual pathway. This would mask a disease association.

■ The measurement of the **exposure(s)** must be collected in a comparable way for cases and controls. Exposure information can be collected via an interview or questionnaire. This is a simple and quick technique, but it may be adversely affected by the ability of subjects to recall historical exposures, where cases have more vested interests in recalling the exposures than controls, and sometimes rely on 'proxy' respondents, e.g. carers, or parents of children. Other approaches to collecting information on exposure are depended on historical records, where obvious disadvantage is that records can be inaccurate, incomplete and were not originally collected for the study purposes. And, if possible, the exposure information can come from collecting biological markers of exposure.

■ The analysis of a case-control study involves comparing the odds of exposure among cases to the odds of exposure among controls. This contrast typically is presented as an OR, and it has a scale of measurement analogous to that of a risk ratio or rate ratio, with the null value of 1 and risk increasing exposures having values greater than 1 and risk lowering exposures having values less than 1. The further the point estimate of the OR is from 1, the stronger the association. Statistical precision of the estimate is reflected in the width of CIs around the point estimate.

(Lijian Lei   Jintao Wang)

STUDY QUESTIONS

1. *Please compare the difference and relationship of cohort study and case-control study.*
2. *How can you match cases and controls in case-control study?*
3. *What are the advantages and disadvantages of case control studies?*

IMPORTANT TERMINOLOGY

cohort study	队列研究
case-control study	病例对照研究
sample	样本
observational epidemiological study	观察性流行病学研究
source population	源人群
risk factor	危险因素
random sample	随机样本
matching	匹配
confounding	混杂
frequency matching	频数匹配
group matching	成组匹配
individual matching	个体匹配
categorical variable	分类变量
continuous variable	连续变量
exposure	暴露
bias	偏倚
biomarker	生物标志物
odds ratio (OR)	比值比
confidence interval	可信区间

FURTHER READING

Rothman KJ, Greenland S, Timothy LL. Modern epidemiology. 3rd edition. Lippincott Williams & Wilkins. 2008.

Ahrens W, Pigeot I. Handbook of Epidemiology. Bremen Institute for Prevention Research and Social Medicine (BIPS). Berlin, Germany. 2006; 474-477.

Marshall T. What is a case-control study. International Journal of Epidemiology 2004; 33: 612-617.

REFERENCES

Darby SC,Ewertz M,McGale P, et al. Risk of ischemic heart disease in women after radiotherapy for breast cancer. *N Engl J Med. 2013,368(11): 987-998.*

Porta M. A dictionary of epidemiology. 5th. edition. New York: Oxford University Press, 2008. ISBN 978-0-19-531450-2 and ISBN 0-19-531450-6 [1] (the 6th. was published in June 2014).

Early Breast Cancer Trialists' Collaborative Group. Effects of radiotherapy and of differences in the extent of surgery for early breast cancer on local recurrence and on 15-year survival: an overview of the randomised trials. *Lancet,* 2005; 366: 2087-2106.

D'Souza G, Kreimer AR, Viscidi R, et al. Case–Control Study of HumanPapillomavirus and Oropharyngeal Cancer. *The New England Journal of Medicine.* 2007; 356; 1944-1956.

Clinical Trials

HEALTH SCENARIO

Stroke is a potentially debilitating medical event that affects approximately 17 million people worldwide each year, leaving more than 30% of survivors permanently disabled. Given this impact, there is great demand for treatments that significantly improve functional outcome after a stroke. To date, few clinical trials for the treatment of acute stroke have succeeded. Suppose you and a team of collaborators have a new treatment that you would like to test for use in patients who have had strokes. Where do you begin? How many patients do you need to sample to know if your treatment is safe and effective? How do you choose a comparison group and allocate treatment? How do you choose the outcome of interest and conduct the analysis of your data? These questions will be addressed in the following sections.

INTRODUCTION

A clinical trial is a prospective research study conducted in humans to assess the impact of an experimental intervention. The intervention can be a drug product, a device such as a surgical stent or diagnostic tool, a procedure such as a surgical treatment, or a behavioral intervention. **Clinical trials** are a critical step to therapeutic development because they provide the necessary methodology to make inferences with minimal bias and the best possible precision. Clinical trials have been in existence since the 1700s, although the primary concepts and terminology of trials were not identified until much later (**Figure 7-1**, Timeline), and clinical trial methods and regulations

continue to be developed.

The history of clinical trials is important for understanding the impetus for good clinical practice guidelines, as well as the evolution of the drug and device development process. On average, the typical time from initial development to introduction into clinical practice for a drug in the United States is 15 years (Woosley and Cossman, 2007). Because therapeutic development is a time-consuming and costly process, it is important to take the time to develop the most appropriate study design and ensure proper conduct and analysis of the trial. There are plenty of examples of failed clinical trials, and the cause is not necessarily the absence of a treatment effect. For example, several trials were conducted in acute stroke only to conclude that patients may not have been treated early enough after the injury. Similarly, hundreds of AIDS trials were conducted before it was determined that CD4 cell levels might not be a reliable surrogate for AIDS. There are examples in areas where technology is evolving quickly in which the intervention under study becomes outdated by the end of the trial. Some of these failures can be avoided with the appropriate trial design.

A successful trial depends not only on the right design but also on the right team. Clinical trials demand a team approach, which includes, at a minimum, the epidemiologist, clinical researcher, biostatistician, study coordinator, and patients. This chapter provides an introductory view of clinical trials, including study design, study population, randomization and blinding methods, sample size estimation, and outcomes and analyses.

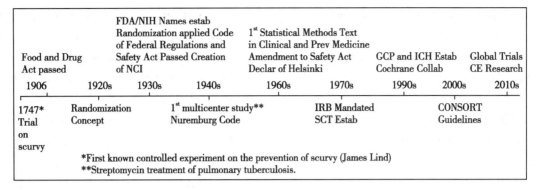

Figure 7-1. Clinical trial history. CE, Comparative Effectiveness; CFR, Code of Federal Regulations; CONSORT,Consolidated Standards of Reporting Trials; FDA, Food and Drug Administration; GCP, Good Clinical Practice; ICH,International Conference on Harmonization; IRB, Institutional Review Board; NCI, National Cancer Institute; NIH,National Institutes of Health; SCT, Society for Clinical Trials.

CLINICAL TRIAL DESIGNS

There are a variety of clinical trial designs. The best design for any specific study depends on a number of issues, including the research question to be addressed, the type of treatment under investigation, and characteristics of the patient population being studied. Although we often think of clinical trials as a method for investigating new therapeutic interventions, clinical trials can also investigate prevention strategies, screening and diagnostic efforts, or supportive care designed to lessen symptom severity and improve quality of life rather than to cure disease.

Sound scientific clinical investigation almost always requires that a control group be used against which the experimental intervention can be compared. To control for expectations and some of the "nonspecific" therapeutic benefit of contact with professionals, many medication trials use a **placebo**, *a biologically inactive substance that is identical in appearance to the medication under investigation.* In trials of therapeutic devices, there is usually some attempt made to mimic the device application while not delivering the therapeutic elements of treatment (e.g., sham transcranial magnetic stimulation in which the device is applied but no current is delivered). In some disease states, the use of a placebo is considered unethical because there are known efficacious therapies and to deny a participant access to these treatments places them at unnecessary risk for harm. In these cases, an active control group receiv-

ing an existing standard treatment typically is used.

As recently as 50 years ago, the primary means of evaluating a new treatment was to compare a group of individuals treated with the new method to outcomes observed in the past from a group of individuals who received standard therapy, referred to as "historical controls." There are several problems inherent in this approach. The primary problem is that it does not allow the investigator to control for the effects of important potential prognostic characteristics of the groups over time (e.g., age, sex, socioeconomic factors). In addition, there could be important variations in the disease state depending on seasonal variation, changes in environmental determinants, and so on over time. In addition, diagnostic criteria and sensitivity of methods for diagnosis of various disease states may change over time, making historical controls a less valid comparison group. For example, improved detection methods may result in earlier stage, more treatable extent of disease than existed historically.

As such, a randomized, controlled clinical trial is often considered to be the "gold standard" for testing a new medication or therapeutic device. Other common designs include pre-/post-, crossover and factorial (**Figure 7-2**). These are generally conducted using a **parallel group design** in which two or more treatment groups are treated at approximately the same time and directly compared (**Figure 7-2**). In a pre-post comparison study design, individuals serve as their own controls with a basic comparison made before and after treatment. In a **cross-over study** design, *each participant also serves as his or her own control, but subjects are randomized to sequences of treatments.* For example, at random, half of subjects receive treatment A followed by treatment B, and the other half at random receive treatment B followed by treatment A. Varying the order in which the subjects receive the treatment allows for investigation of whether there is any impact of the order in which the treatments are delivered on the treatment outcome. A "wash-out" period or time between treatment periods is also often used to minimize the likelihood that the treatment in the first period will impact the outcomes of the treatment in the second period ("**carry-over effect**"). A cross-over design study can have more than two treatment periods. There are several advantages to the cross-over design. Because each subject is used as his or her own control, the treatment comparison has only within-subject variability compared with between-subject variability, allowing a smaller sample size to be studied. There are, however, a number of disadvantages. It is most suitable for studying chronic conditions (e.g., diabetes mellitus) that can be expected to return to a baseline level of severity at the beginning of the second treatment period and is not a suitable design for the study of any disease states that may be cured during the first treatment period (e.g., many acute infections). In addition, the assumption that the effects of intervention during the first period will not carry over into subsequent periods must be valid. In addition, subject drop-out (i.e., voluntarily or involuntarily discontinuing participation) before the second treatment period can severely limit the validity of the results.

The **factorial design** (**Figure 7-2**) attempts to *evaluate two interventions compared with a control within a single trial.* Given the cost and effort involved in recruitment for clinical trials, this is an efficient and attractive proposition. If it can be validly assumed that there is no interaction between the two interventions being compared, with only a modest increase in sample size, two experiments can be conducted simultaneously. However, one concern with factorial design is the possibility of an interaction between the two interventions being compared. An **interaction** exists *when the two treatments administered together have a less or greater effect than would be expected from the combination of the separate effects of the treatments when administered individually.* An interaction may arise when the two treatments impact on different biological processes, thereby amplifying each other's effect. When interaction is present, the sample size must be increased to account for the interaction. As such, the factorial design can be particularly appropriate and efficient either when there is no interaction expected or when the interaction between two treatments is an important focus of the study.

Other types of designs include cluster randomized trials, equivalence trials and adaptive trials. These designs address a specific study setting as described herein. In group allocation or **cluster randomization** designs, *a group of individuals (e.g., those attending a clinic, school, or community) is randomized to a particular intervention or control.* In this type of design, the basic sampling unit is the group, not individual participants, and the overall sample size needs be inflated accordingly. Cluster randomized designs are a good option when one is con-

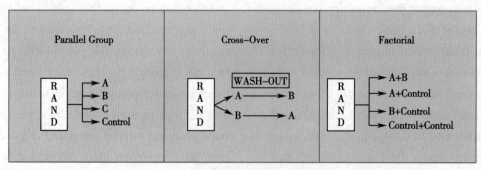

Figure 7-2. Study design examples.

cerned with contamination across treatment groups. For example, a trial on a new educational program should be concerned with **contamination** (*those not intended to have the experimental treatment receiving it inadvertently because of proximity and sharing with the experimental subjects*) within the same school or same grades. Therefore, one would consider randomizing by grades or schools rather than by individual students.

In studies of **equivalency, or noninferiority trials,** *the objective is to test whether a new intervention is as good as or no worse than an established one.* The control or standard therapy in such a trial must have established efficacy. The investigator must specify what is meant by equivalence because it cannot be proven that two therapies have absolutely identical effects, as an infinite sample size would be required to prove equivalence. In this situation, outcomes other than the primary become important as frequency, and severity of adverse events (AEs), quality of life measures, ease of use, and costs may be important secondary bases of comparison in preferring one treatment over another.

An **adaptive design** *allows predefined design adaptations to be made to trial procedures of ongoing clinical trials.* In adaptive trials, as the trial progresses, the collected data are used to guide the predefined adaptation of the trial during its progress. The adaptations can be to drop a treatment arm that is not effective, alter dose levels, or increase the trial size if pretrial assumptions are not as predicted. This means that the dosing, eligibility criteria, sample size, or treatment settings can be adjusted during the course of the trial as evidence accumulates. The most important aspect of these designs is that the adaptations must be defined before the onset of the trial so that the statistical team can assess the impact of the changes on trial operating characteristics such as sample size and the possibility of a false conclusion. Adaptive designs have the potential to accelerate therapeutic development, but there are methodologic and implementation challenges in terms of randomization and statistical analysis that are specific to adaptive design clinical trials.

One of the motivations for conducting clinical trials is the persistent and unexplained variability in clinical practice and high rates of care for which evidence of effectiveness is lacking. The increasing cost of health care has fueled an increasing demand for evidence of clinical effectiveness. *Clinical trials that are developed specifically to answer the questions faced by clinical decision makers* are called **pragmatic** or **practical clinical trials** (PCTs). PCTs often address practical questions about the risks, benefits, and costs of interventions as would occur in routine clinical practice. In general, PCTs focus on a relatively easily administered intervention and an easily ascertained outcome. Characteristic features of PCTs are that they compare clinically relevant alternative interventions, include a diverse population of study participants, recruit from heterogeneous practice settings, and collect data on a broad range of health outcomes (Tunis et al., 2003).

CLINICAL TRIAL PHASES

Clinical studies conducted to evaluate the therapeutic potential of a compound for a given illness have been divided into four phases. Before clinical studies, one often begins with translational research that brings the laboratory bench science and preclinical studies to the bedside so that new interventions (e.g., drugs, devices, behavioral interventions) can be further studied to develop promising new treatments. Clinical studies generally begin cautiously. As experience with the agent grows, the questions expand from tolerable dose to safety and then to efficacy. The number of subjects studied at each phase and the duration of studies can vary significantly depending on statistical considerations, the prevalence of the disease under consideration, and the agent under investigation. There are, however, some general principles and procedures regarding the four phases of clinical testing described below.

Phase I Clinical Trials

In **phase I trials,** *the compound under investigation is administered to humans for the first time.* Phase I studies generally are conducted in a hospital setting with close medical monitoring. When possible, phase I studies are conducted in normal, healthy volunteers to allow for the evaluation of the effects of the drug in a subject with no preexisting disease conditions. In some situations when it is not ethical to use normal human volunteers (e.g., testing oncology drugs, which are highly toxic), testing may be done in volunteers who have the disorder under investigation and have exhausted all other available treatment options.

The purpose of a phase I trial is to determine basic safety, pharmacokinetic, and pharmacologic information. These studies generally share certain characteristics. A series of ascending dose levels is used, with initial doses determined by extrapolation from animal data, beginning with a low dose and proceeding until a dose range suitable for use in later trials is identified. A small group of subjects is treated concurrently and may receive one dose of medication or several doses in a series of consecutive treatment periods. Data from each set of studies are generally collected and assessed before choosing the next set of doses for administration. Adverse Events (AEs) are investigated intensively in phase I trials. In some cases, such as the investigation of oncology drugs, dose escalation is continued until limited by toxicity for the determination of a maximally tolerated dose (MTD). Although clinical monitoring for AEs is one of the critical elements of all first-in-human studies, the MTD is not the universal endpoint of phase I investigation, and when appropriate, the endpoint for dose escalation may be a given plasma concentration or a biomarker for some indication of the action for the agent (Collins, 2000).

A diversity of procedures can be used in phase I trials. For many compounds, it is anticipated that AEs will not be a major limiting concern. In this case, AEs are monitored, but the principal observations of interest are pharmacokinetic and pharmacodynamic endpoints. Parameters repeatedly assessed during most phase I trials include vital signs, physical and neurologic status, laboratory testing (in particular hepatic, renal, hematopoietic function), cardiac conduction (serial electrocardiography [ECG] or telem-

etry), and AEs. Pharmacokinetic parameters after single, repeated, and a range of doses are assessed. Assessments include maximal plasma concentrations, time to maximal plasma concentration, time to steady state, elimination half-life, plasma accumulation, and total drug exposure to test for dose-plasma level proportionality. Studies investigating bioavailability, particularly by the oral route of administration, food effects on absorption, and relative bioavailability studies of different formulations (e.g., capsule and solution), are also conducted. The metabolic profile and elimination pathways also are determined.

Phase II Clinical Trials

Phase II clinical trials range from small, single-arm studies to randomized trials comparing a control treatment with the experimental drug in either a single dose or at several doses. Because these studies vary considerably in size and study objectives, the study designs are quite heterogeneous. In phase II studies, the study subjects are the patient population that has the disorder of interest. *There is an assessment of treatment efficacy as well as safety.* Phase II trials are designed to extend the safety database and provide initial evidence for efficacy of the compound. Phase II trials are not designed to give definitive evidence of efficacy, and the goal of the trial is to lead to a decision concerning further (phase III) testing rather than regulatory submission. Although the focus of a phase II study is efficacy, further information about drug delivery, protocol feasibility, dosing, and AEs are gathered. As in phase I, data collected may include pharmacokinetics, repeated physical and neurologic examinations, comprehensive laboratory testing, cardiac conduction (ECG), and vital signs. The primary outcome variables typically are focused on the target condition. These usually include relevant illness appropriate rating scales such as the Clinical Global Impression (CGI) rating for mental health studies, the modified Rankin scale (mRS) for stroke, and so forth. There is an emphasis on adverse effects and compliance, usually determined by both pill count and pharmacokinetic parameters. Frequency of visits depends on the target condition and the agent under investigation. There may be a required period of "in-clinic," close medical assessment after administration of the initial dose (s) of the compound in situations when there are some acute effects of concern.

Phase III Clinical Trials

Phase III trials *are large clinical studies that can involve the treatment of several hundred subjects from multiple centers with a goal of assessing therapeutic benefit.* The large number of patients involved allows for the development of a broad database of information about the safety and efficacy of the drug candidate. Despite the large numbers of patients studied, the exclusion criteria for phase III trials are stringent. As in phase II trials, subjects with comorbid conditions other than the target condition under investigation generally are excluded.

Study designs used in phase III trials are less heterogeneous than those used in phase II because of the need to meet defined regulatory standards for the New Drug Application (NDA) to the Food and Drug Administration (FDA). The study duration is variable depending on the therapeutic area. The assessments of laboratory data and physical and neurologic examination are less frequent than in the phase I and II trials and outcome measures generally include assessment of the primary outcome (target condition) using disease-specific measures (e.g., reducing symptoms, arresting or reversing an underlying pathologic process, decreasing complications of the illness) and secondary outcome measures such as quality of life and disability measures.

Phase III trials often include fixed-dose studies, flexible dose studies, and studies that include the comparison of a "gold standard" treatment along with the experimental agent and placebo. The large group of geographically and demographically diverse participants may allow for the identification of rare AEs that only affect a few patients. Despite the earlier testing, approximately one in five potential drugs are eliminated during phase III of testing. However, if a drug candidate is successful in phase I and II, some

of the phase III studies will be "pivotal" studies that will serve as the basis for FDA approval.

Phase IV Clinical Trials

Phase IV trials are initiated after a drug has been approved by the FDA. These trials are also referred to as post-marketing studies. *They are generally conducted for the approved indication, but they may evaluate different doses, the effects of extended therapy, or the safety of the agent in patient populations that were not studied in the premarketing clinical trials.* Phase IV trials may be initiated by the sponsor in an attempt to gather more information on the safety and efficacy of the drug, or they may be requested by the FDA. To evaluate the risk of rare side effects, phase IV trials often involve very large and diverse study populations.

STUDY PARTICIPANT SELECTION

The study population is a subset of individuals with the condition or characteristics of interest as defined by study eligibility criteria. The types of characteristics typically used for eligibility criteria include stage or severity of illness, age and gender of patients, absence of other comorbid conditions, and ease of follow-up. Careful consideration of study eligibility criteria is essential because it will impact the generalizability (extent to which results can be extrapolated to other patients) and utility of the study. In general, eligibility criteria are related to participant safety and the anticipated effect of the intervention. If the study population is very homogeneous with highly selective inclusion and exclusion criteria, the decreased variability in response means that a treatment effect is more likely to be detected if one truly exists. However, with a narrowly defined study population, the study results will not be as easily generalized to the entire universe of individuals with the disease state in question. However, if the study population is heterogeneous with few exclusion criteria, the variability in response may make it more difficult to discern a treatment effect, but the results of the study will have broad generalizability. It is of critical importance that the investigators give a careful and detailed description of the study population so that readers can fully assess the applicability of the findings to their patient populations. When defining the eligibility criteria, it is important to consider who will potentially benefit from the proposed experimental intervention, who will have minimal risk, and who will adhere to the intervention.

Choosing the right study population is important; however, it is just as important to ensure that certain populations are not neglected or coerced to participate and that there is an equitable selection of participants. For example, in the history of clinical research, it has been argued that women, children, and disadvantaged ethnic groups have either been harmfully neglected or exploited in clinical studies. These populations are referred to as *vulnerable populations*, a category of participants subject to an inequity in research. This category includes children, prisoners, pregnant women, disadvantaged ethnic groups, and persons with physical or mental disabilities. Great care should be taken when designing a clinical trial to ensure minimal risk to the participating population and equity in participant selection. This is why clinical research has a participant consent process referred to as the *informed consent* process. One main requirement when conducting a clinical trial is that all participants are fully informed about the trial. This includes understanding the intervention they may be given, what they will have to do if they take part in the trial, what benefit they might gain or what harm may come to them, what will happen to them after the trial is over, and what their rights may be to other treatments. When obtaining consent from minors or mentally impaired populations, there must be a person who is permitted to give consent on the participant's behalf such as a parent or a legally authorized representative.

RANDOMIZATION AND BLINDING

Randomization of study participants is a key component of clinical trials with multiple treatment arms. *The goal of randomization is to establish comparable groups with respect to both known and unknown prognostic factors, to minimize selection and accidental biases, and to ensure that appropriate statistical tests have valid significance levels.* An important question regards how to randomize. Several randomization methods are available. Fixed allocation schemes, including simple randomization, **blocked randomization**, and **stratified randomization,** assign the intervention with a prespecified probability (equal or unequal) that remains constant during the study period. **Simple randomization** is analogous to flipping a coin when the rules are prespecified (e.g., heads = experimental; tails = control). Although easy to implement and provides random treatment assignment, simple randomization does not take into account important prognostic variables, so the balance of these variables across treatment arms is not guaranteed.

Constrained randomization, which includes blocked and stratified schemes, addresses this potential limitation of simple randomization. Using a blocked scheme, randomization is done within small subsets (small blocks). Block size is determined by the number of treatment arms and must be an exact integer multiple of the number of arms. For example, if a trial with two treatment arms has a chosen block size of four, then there are six possible permutations of treatments (ABAB, AABB, and so on). A list of blocks can be pre-generated, and when enrollment begins, blocks are randomly selected. It is important to completely fill a block before using another block because complete blocks ensure balance in treatment assignments. Although blocking does not ensure balance of important prognostic factors, this can be achieved by adding stratification. For example, if gender impacts the outcome of interest, the researcher should ensure that males and females receive equal treatment assignments. In a blocked stratified scheme, blocks would be set up within each stratum (i.e., male, female) to provide treatment assignment balance within each stratum. Although blocked, stratified schemes have been used commonly in trials (mainly because of their ease of implementation); there are cons to this approach. Specifically, one loses randomness in the assignment as a block fills, and the assignment becomes deterministic by the end of a block. As randomization methodologies expand, there are alternatives to fixed and constrained allocation schemes such as **adaptive randomization** schemes. Adaptive schemes allocate patients with a changing probability and include number adaptive, baseline adaptive, and response (outcome) adaptive. Although the various adaptive schemes can be more complex to implement, the advantages include minimized deterministic assignments and maintenance of the randomness of assignments. Schemes include minimization, minimal sufficient balance, and play the winner.

In addition to randomization, **blinding**, *which means keeping the identity of treatment assignment hidden*, is another important aspect of a clinical trial design. In a **single-blinded study**, the treatment assignment is unknown to the patients; in a **double-blinded study**, the treatment assignment is unknown either to the patients or to their treating physicians or the assessors who decide the outcome; in a **triple-blinded study**, neither patients, physicians, and assessors, nor the assigners of the treatment and the persons who manipulate data analysis (analysts) know the assignment. In a double-or triple-blinded study, the treatment assignment may be revealed to the patient and physician if there are serious or unexpected side effects. Although not always feasible, blinding has several important features. It minimizes the potential biases resulting from differences in patient management, treatment, or interpretation of results and the influence of patient expectation, and it avoids subjective assessment and decisions that could occur if investigators or participants are aware of the treatment assignment.

Ideally, the participant, investigator, and evaluation team should be blinded to the treatment allocation, and it is important to ensure that the treatment assignment information remains confidential until the end of the trial. For example, if a participant is made aware that the next treatment assignment is to a placebo control arm, then he or she may decline participation, which may lead to a selection bias in the study population. If the investigator is made aware of the next treatment assignment, then he or she may decide to not enroll the next patient because of a specific patient characteristic such as disease severity, which also could produce selection bias. Similarly, if the various parties are blind to treatment allocation but are made aware after the assignment, then they may withdraw consent, or the care of that participant may be impacted if the evaluating team knows what intervention the patient received.

As previously mentioned, blinding is not always feasible. When considering the feasibility of blinding, ethics and practicality must be examined. The investigator needs to ensure that implementation of a blinding scheme will not result in harm to the participants. In terms of practicality, surgical trials, diagnostic studies, and behavioral studies often struggle with implementing blinding because the person delivering the intervention knows the assignment. Blinding of the allocation can still be maintained; however, at a minimum, the post-intervention evaluation should be done by a person(s) who is (are) blind to individual treatment assignment.

SAMPLE SIZE ESTIMATION

For every clinical trial, sample size must be determined to ensure adequate statistical power (ability to discern an effect, if present) for the proposed analysis plan. The question that is answered by sample size estimation is, "How many participants are needed in order to ensure a certain probability of detecting a clinically relevant difference at a defined significance level?" The overall goal of sample size estimation is to achieve reasonable precision in estimating the outcome of interest. That is to say, one should characterize the treatment effect within an acceptably narrow range of values consistent with the data. The study sample size should reflect what is needed to address the primary objective of the trial and the analysis of the outcome and should be enough to examine the secondary outcomes. Just as important, sample size needs to be determined so that a budget can be derived. The estimation of study sample size starts with the primary outcome. One needs to define the quantitative measure (outcome) and determine how to analyze it in order to estimate sample size. When there is a dichotomous (yes/no) outcome from a paired sample (McNemar test) but the sample size is estimated for an independent outcome (chi-square test), an incorrect sample size will be estimated and the trial is threatened to be underpowered to detect the relevant differences.

When calculating sample size, four parameters need to be predefined: the probability of a type I error, the probability of a type II error, the standard deviation of the outcome measure, and what you determine to be the clinically relevant difference between the experimental intervention and the control intervention. The type I error occurs when a null hypothesis is falsely rejected (false-positive); for example, when testing to see if the experimental intervention is superior to the control intervention, a type I error occurs when there is a false claim of superiority. The probability of a type I error is referred to as the significance level of a test. Common values for a significant level are 0.05 or 0.10. A type II error occurs when one fails to reject the null hypothesis (e.g., in the superiority setting, this is falsely claiming no difference when in fact a true difference exists, false-negative). Common values for type II error probabilities are 0.10 and 0.20. One minus type II error is the statistical power of the trial.

Clinical trials are concerned about power because the statistical power of the test tells us how likely we are to reject the null hypothesis given that the alternative hypothesis is true. If the power is too low (<80%), then we have insufficient chance of detecting the predefined clinically relevant difference. Invariably, the cause of low power is inadequate sample size. Just as important, though, is that we must acknowledge that statistical significance does not imply clinical significance. With unlimited funds, one could have a large enough study to have adequate power to detect a difference that is so small that it does not have any clinical meaning. For example, if one could afford to conduct a 10,000-patient trial

and detected less than 1-point change in a continuous outcome scale, there is reason to doubt whether that 1-point change is clinically meaningful. Will the difference detected change practice? That is the most important question for the clinical researcher to bring to the table for sample size estimation.

The clinically relevant difference for trials is either defined as the absolute difference or the relative difference between the experimental treatment and control (i.e., how much difference should there be in order to change practice). In trials for acute spinal cord injury, the primary outcome is often the mean American Spinal Injury Association (ASIA) motor score at 12 months after randomization. When estimating sample size for a two-arm trial, we turn to the literature on the ASIA motor score for this population to guide us in determining the expected 12-month mean ASIA motor score for standard of care. If we assume that the control arm (standard of care) is going to have a mean score of 25 with a standard deviation of 15, then we need to determine what absolute difference should be detected in order to state the experimental treatment is beneficial compared with control. This is not an easy task and requires a combination of literature review, clinical expertise, and consensus. This is similar when the outcome is a proportion. Consider a trial with a primary outcome of proportion of successes in which success is defined by a certain predefined threshold of improvement. If we assume the proportion of successes in the population that is receiving the control is 30%, then how much better (e.g., 40%, 50%) does the proportion need to be in the experimental arm in order to claim it is better? This can be defined in absolute or relative terms. On an absolute scale, we can state that the experimental arm must have at least an absolute increase of 30%. We can take that same difference and turn it into a relative scale; the experimental arm must have a 50% relative increase in the success rate compared with the control. Both are acceptable approaches to defining the clinically relevant difference, but it is important to be clear which scale you are basing your sample size calculations on because you can get very different results if you mistakenly used the 50% absolute difference rather than the intended 30%.

OUTCOMES AND ANALYSIS

Research studies start with a question, which leads to study objectives, which lead to the definition of outcomes. Researchers often have multiple questions, and it is the responsibility of the study team to determine the primary versus the secondary and tertiary questions. The reason to delineate the major hypothesis is because in clinical trials, the primary question drives the various aspects of the study design, including sample size, study population, study procedures, and data analyses. Consider common questions in a clinical trial setting: What dose of a new experimental anticlotting drug is safe and well tolerated in patients with thrombotic strokes? Is an innovative surgical stenting procedure safe and effective in patients with carotid artery blockages? Is another new drug showing a signal of efficacy in preventing strokes in patients with transient ischemic attacks? These questions lead to objectives: to determine safety, to determine dose, and to determine efficacy. After one has the question and objectives, then one can determine the outcomes that need to be measured.

Outcomes, also referred to as endpoints, *are the quantitative measures that correspond to the study objectives.* The outcome can be continuous, categorical, ordinal, nominal, or a time to an event, or the outcome can be a composite measure. When choosing the study outcome, it is desirable for the outcome to have the following properties: valid and reliable, capable of being observed for every trial participant, free of measurement error, and clinically relevant. All of these properties are important, and the combination of the literature and the features of the disease that the intervention is targeting to improve should be used to help decide the best outcomes for the clinical trial. For example, in acute spinal cord injury trials, researchers examine mean ASIA motor scores to interpret treatment effects. For oncology trials, a common study outcome is a time to event

such as overall survival or time to tumor progression. In acute stroke and cardiovascular disease trials, the outcome often is a proportion of good or bad outcomes as defined by dichotomizing the modified Rankin scale for stroke and reporting the proportion of nonfatal myocardial infarctions or the total mortality rate for cardiovascular disease. After the outcomes are defined, then one can consider the analysis plan.

If the primary outcome is a categorical variable, then an appropriate analysis for categorical outcomes must be used. For example, a simple dichotomous outcome (e.g., success or failure; yes or no) could be analyzed using a chi-square test. If a cell size is small, however, then the analysis may use Fisher's exact test, or if data are not independent (e.g., each participant receives both treatment A and treatment B), then McNemar's test for paired data should be used. **Table 7-1** provides an example of how to display the data for a dichotomous outcome. When reporting results from a trial, it is very important to report both the point estimate of the treatment effect with the appropriate confidence interval (CI) and the P value produced from the statistical test. The CI includes the range of values that are consistent with the data observed at a defined level of statistical precision (e.g., 95%). This information will give the audience a more complete picture of the benefit of the experimental treatment. For example, based on the data in **Table 7-1**, we see that the experimental arm had 34 successes out of 141 randomized into that arm (proportion of success, p_e, of 0.24), and the control arm had 25 successes out of 141 randomizations ($p_c = 0.18$). The treatment effect of this trial can be reported as a 6% absolute risk difference (0.24 − 0.18) with a 95% CI of −3.1%, 15.8% between the proportion of success in the experimental arm compared with the control arm. This point estimate can be supported by conducting a chi-square test and reporting a test statistic of 1.74 and a P value of 0.19. Note that the 95% CI included the value of no effect (0% difference). This tells us that the point estimate of 6% difference is not statistically significant at the 5% level ($P > 0.05$). In other words, we cannot exclude chance as an explanation for treatment differences of this magnitude with a sample of this size.

Table 7-1 Results of a hypothetical trial concerning the 12-month outcome of success or failure in patients with the targeted disease

	Treatment		
	Experimental	**Control**	**Total**
Success	34	25	59
Failure	107	116	223
Total	141	141	282

Alternative approaches of reporting the treatment effect include percentage absolute risk reduction (or benefit), relative risk or number needed to treat (NNT), which is the number of patients needed to be treated with the experimental treatment rather than the control treatment for one additional patient to benefit. Using the data in **Table 7-1**, we can calculate these measures as follows:

Percent absolute risk reduction or benefit

$$= \frac{P_e - P_c}{P_c} \times 100\% = \frac{(34/141 - 25/141)}{25/141}$$

$$\times 100\% = 36\%$$

This means that the experimental group had about a one third improvement in response likelihood compared with the baseline response among controls.

$$\text{Risk ratio} = \frac{P_e}{P_c} = \frac{0.241}{0.177} = 1.36$$

This means that the likelihood of a successful response was 36% higher within the experimental group when compared with the control group.

$$\text{NNT} = 1/\text{ARR} = \frac{1}{0.241 - 0.177} = 15.7$$

Where ARR is the Absolute Risk Reduction. This means that almost 16 patients need to be treated with the experimental method in order to have one more patient respond than would otherwise.

All of these summary measures are acceptable for reporting clinical trial data. For this particular example, the measures should be interpreted as follows: being treated with the experimental therapy provides about one third more successful outcomes than the control therapy, the risk of having a beneficial (successful) outcome in the experimental treatment group is about one third greater than in the control group, and the experimental treatment will lead to one more success for every 16 patients treated. Choosing which metric to report is a decision that should be based on what the study team believes is most important for their audience to know in order to understand the magnitude of the treatment effect. Sometimes a combination of the measures is provided. In addition to these various point estimates, the reported value should be accompanied by a two-sided CI to show the uncertainty in the estimate. Although the point estimate tells us something about the treatment effect, the point estimate alone does not provide information on whether this value is statistically different from no effect. By including the CI, we are providing valuable information on the statistical precision of our estimate. For example, the risk ratio is 1.36 in the above example and has a 95% CI of 0.86, 2.16. A risk ratio of 1 indicates that there is no difference between the two treatments ($P_e = P_c$) and as it moves away from 1 we begin to see greater differences in outcomes between the groups. The CI provides a range of plausible values for the risk ratio, and because the interval includes 1, we can conclude that there is no statistical difference (at $P < 0.05$) between the two treatment arms. A similar approach can be seen with the reported interval for the absolute risk reduction (ARR) or benefit. In that scenario, an interval that contains zero indicates no risk difference between the two treatment arms ($p_e = p_c$).

Often clinical trial analyses include a known *prognostic variable*, a variable that impacts outcome regardless of treatment. For example, in certain acute neurologic diseases such as stroke, traumatic brain injury, and spinal cord injury, the baseline severity of the injury impacts outcome such that more severe cases tend to have worse functional outcomes. The analysis for these outcomes often includes an adjustment for baseline severity to account for the impact of severity on outcome because our true focus is the impact of treatment on outcome regardless of severity. The treatment effect within each subgroup of severity may be of secondary interest; however, the study often lacks sufficient statistical power for subgroup analysis. Overall, if the incorrect analysis method is used, then correct inferences about treatment effect cannot be made, and the trial will lack validity. **Table 7-2** provides a basic guide for analysis choices.

In addition to choosing the correct analysis, it is important to analyze the correct population. In randomized clinical trials, the primary analysis should be conducted on the intent-to-treat population, which is defined by the randomization assignment. If a participant was randomized to receive the experimental treatment and it is known that he or she ended up never receiving it, that participant should still be analyzed as part of the experimental arm. Although this may seem illogical at first, the intent-to-treat population is a more unbiased representation of the population with the disease being studied. The reason it is less biased is that there are several scenarios in which a participant may not receive the assigned treatment, including clinical errors and participant choice if the experimental treatment has negative side effects or if the participant forgets to take the treatment or drops out of the study. Not receiving the experimental therapy can be similar, in some situations, to being in the control arm. We do not want to analyze the data by moving those individuals to the control arm, however, because then we lose the benefits of randomization as described earlier. In addition, these scenarios can occur outside of

the trial in the general population with the disease. When we interpret results from a trial, particularly a phase III definitive trial, we want the results to be generalizable to patients outside of the trial. Accordingly, it is recommended to be conservative in the estimate of a treatment effect and report the results using the intent-to-treat population.

Another important aspect of outcomes and analysis is the handling of missing data. In clinical trials, missing outcome data is to be expected. Study participants may miss a follow-up visit, may withdraw consent, or may move and be unable to be followed for the remainder of the study. All of these scenarios can contribute to missing data, which impacts the data analysis. As mentioned earlier, in an intent-to-treat analysis, we would not remove participants with missing outcome data from the analysis. Instead, we have to keep them in the analysis population in order to reduce the potential bias of our treatment estimate. There are several methods for imputing data for missing observations, but this is beyond the scope of this chapter. The overall goal in the design and conduct of a trial is to minimize the amount of missing data by ensuring that outcomes of interest can be measured in all participants, the length of participant follow-up is reasonable, and there is frequent contact with the participants throughout the follow-up period.

One other point to consider is categorizing a continuous endpoint. Although dichotomous outcomes

Table 7-2 Outcomes and common analyses

Data Type	Examples	Common Tests for Differences
Categorical	Nominal, dichotomous, and nondichotomous—success or failure, present or absent, nationalities	Test for binomial proportions (one sample or two independent samples) Chi-square test (independent data) McNemar's test (matched paired data) Sign test (nonparametric)
Ordinal	Values that have a natural ordering (e.g., dislike, neutral, like); rating of 1 to 5	Trend test Sign-rank test (nonparametric paired samples) Rank sum test (nonparametric independent samples)
Continuous	Comparison of means or medians	Student's t-test (one sample or two independent samples) Paired t-test (two dependent samples) Rank sum test (non-normal data) ANOVA (more than two independent samples) Sign-rank test (nonparametric paired samples) Rank sum test (nonparametric independent samples)
Time to event	Comparison of survival curves	Log-rank test

may in some situations provide simplified clinical interpretation, categorization comes with a price. Knowledge of the correct categories is not always available and thus could lead to incorrect results. Caution should be taken when attempting to categorize a continuous outcome. If possible, the existing literature should be reviewed, and the properties of an ideal outcome should be considered.

ETHICAL ISSUES

The investigator who contemplates entering a patient into a randomized clinical trial is faced with several ethical dilemmas. First, is the method of the randomized clinical trial ethically acceptable? One of the most important ethical tenets in medicine is that the patient's welfare is of primary concern, and a caregiver should prescribe the optimal treatment for a patient. It could be argued that even if a clinician has only a hunch or feeling that one treatment is superior, the patient should be offered that treatment. Randomization between two treatments, therefore, might be considered to be unethical. Given the seriousness and possible side effects of medical interventions, however, the axiom "first, do no harm" must always be borne in mind. The history of medicine is replete with examples of treatments now known to be either of no benefit or actually harmful. The clinical trial is considered to be the test method available to determine the benefits and potential harm of treatment regimens.

If the clinical trial method is accepted as appropriate, a decision must be made concerning how to perform trials as ethically as possible. The following is a list of guidelines for medical professionals who are conducting clinical trials:

(1) None of the treatment options included a randomized trial should be known to be inferior to another treatment option based on previous randomized studies, and if a standard treatment regimen exists, it should be used as the control.

(2) The trial should address a question that is of clinical importance and seek to answer the question in a way that will be useful for future patients.

(3) Patients should be told that they are one of a clinical experiment and should be informed in understandable language about all treatment options, the risks and benefits of participation, nature of randomization. The patient who then agrees to participate is said to have given informed consent, which implies that the patient freely chooses to be included in the trial.

(4) The investigators undertaking the trial should be able to recruit in a timely manner the number of patients needed to meet the required sample size.

CONCLUSIONS AND LIMITATIONS

Although clinical trials are an invaluable source of information to drive innovation and improvements in clinical practice, there are a number of challenges facing the clinical research enterprise (Sung et al., 2003). In recent years, there have been concerns expressed over the disconnect between the promise of basic science discovery and the delivery of better health care. This is, in part, due to the failure to translate the findings from clinical trials, often conducted in highly controlled environments, into everyday clinical practice. The reasons for this failure are multifaceted and have led to a new area of research known as implementation and dissemination science. In addition, there are problems with the clinical research environment. It is burdened by rising costs, increasing regulatory controls, and a shortage of qualified investigators and research participants. It is important to engage the public more effectively in clinical research, both as research participants and advocates for research funding. In addition, wider participation of diverse populations in clinical trials will improve the generalizability and applicability of the information gained from the trials. Adaptive trials and PCTs address some of these issues, but there still is a need to develop new clinical trial methodologies and creative approaches to the use of data to examine and improve clinical practice in a timely manner. In addition, efforts to standardize and streamline regulatory processes are critical to improving the efficiency and cost-effectiveness of clinical trials. In conclusion, clinical trials have contributed tremendously to evidence-based clinical practice. Improvements in the approach to clinical trial design and analysis will help to make the information gained through clinical trials even more relevant to efforts to improve clinical practice and health outcomes.

SUMMARY

In summary, a well-designed and conducted clinical trial is essential for therapeutic development. The various clinical trial phases are a gradual progression to addressing the overall question of safety and efficacy. Phase I designs focus on finding the correct dose or treatment regimen to move forward in future studies. Phase II designs focus on further assessment of safety and identifying a signal of efficacy. Phase III designs continue to assess safety and focus on determining efficacy. Phase IV or post-marketing trials further refine safety and efficacy in large clinical populations. There are several study designs to choose from for each trial phase, and the choice should be driven by the primary study question and the goal of reducing biases in order to make correct inferences from the collected data. Features of good trial design include use of a concurrent control group, implementation of randomization and blinding when the design includes two or more treatment arms, a primary outcome that is valid and reliable, sample size estimation that is based on the primary outcome and the clinically relevant difference of interest, and a study population that represents the patient population of interest. In addition to good design, the analysis should complement the design in terms of accounting for the correct variability (e.g., independent vs. paired outcomes) and inclusion of important prognostic variables. The combination of appropriate trial design and analysis promotes unbiased inference of the treatment effect with the best possible precision.

The design and conduct of trials is a team effort composed not only of the clinician but also the statistician, study coordinator, and patients. This chapter introduces readers to key concepts of clinical trials and hopefully provokes further interest in the topic. Clinical trials are quite complex, and design methodology continues to be developed to improve the efficiency of these research studies. The best clinical trial lesson is to become involved in the design and conduct of a trial after becoming familiar with the basic terminology and concepts. Each trial introduces a new lesson on the methodology as well as the practical aspects of conducting a clinical trial.

(Zefang Ren)

IMPORTANT TERMINOLOGY

adaptive design	适应(变化)设计
adaptive randomization	适应(变化)随机化
blocked randomization	整群随机化
carry-over effect	残留效应
clinical trials	临床试验
cross-over study	交叉试验
equivalency trait	等效性试验
non-inferiority trait	非劣效性试验
factorial design	多因素设计
parallel group design	平行设计
phase I/II/III/IV trials	I/II/III/IV 期临床试验
placebo	安慰剂
pragmatic/practical clinical trials (PCTs)	实用性临床试验
simple randomization	简单随机化
single/double/triple-blinding	单盲 / 双盲 / 三盲
stratified randomization	分层随机化

 STUDY QUESTIONS

Questions 1-10: A randomized, double blind, placebo-controlled clinical trial is conducted to determine whether drugs that interfere with the blood clotting effects of platelets can reduce the 2-year risk of a second stroke or death among persons who have had a stroke. Among 1650 persons treated with two antiplatelet drugs, 157 developed a second stroke or died. Among 1650 persons treated with a placebo, 250 developed a second stroke or died.

1. The 2-year risk of a second stroke or death among per-

sons treated with the placebo was

A. 0.095.

B. 0.152.

C. 0.25.

D. 0.63.

E. 1.6.

2. The 2-year risk of a second stroke or death among persons treated with the two antiplatelet drugs was

A. 0.095.

B. 0.152.

C. 0.25.

D. 0.63.

E. 1.6.

3. The risk ratio comparing the 2-year risk of a second stroke or death among persons on antiplatelet therapy to the reference risk among persons treated with the placebo was

A. 0.095.

B. 0.152.

C. 0.25.

D. 0.63.

E. 1.6.

4. With respect to 2-year risk of second stroke or death, the correct interpretation of this study result is that the point estimate for the risk ratio indicates, that two-drug antiplatelet therapy is associated with

A. reduced risk.

B. increased risk.

C. no change in risk.

D. a risk change that cannot be characterized from the information provided.

5. In this study, the treatment groups were similar with regard to baseline characteristics thought to be related to the risk of a second stroke or death. This most likely occurred because of

A. use of a placebo.

B. use of blinding.

C. use of informed consent.

D. use of intention-to-treat analysis.

E. use of randomization.

6. In this study, observer bias was reduced by ensuring that the physicians did not know the treatment assignments of individual patients. This strategy is best described as

A. use of a placebo.

B. use of blinding.

C. use of informed consent.

D. use of intention-to-treat analysis.

E. use of randomization.

7. Subjects in this study were enrolled only after learning about potential risks of receiving antiplatelet therapy. This strategy is best described as

A. use of a placebo.

B. use of blinding.

C. use of informed consent.

D. use of intention-to-treat analysis.

E. use of randomization.

8. Among subjects assigned to antiplatelet therapy, 10% of persons developed bleeding complications and, therefore, antiplatelet medications were discontinued. In the design of this study, however, these persons were still considered as having received antiplatelet therapy. This strategy is best described as

A. use of a placebo.

B. use of blinding.

C. use of informed consent.

D. use of intention-to-treat analysis.

E. use of randomization.

9. In the design of this study, the investigators were willing to accept a 5% likelihood of concluding that antiplatelet therapy reduces risk of second stroke or death, if in truth it is not. The 5% chance is to be described as a(n)

A. alpha level.

B. beta level.

C. statistical power.

D. observe bias.

E. selection bias.

10. A separate, much smaller clinical trial of antiplatelet therapy failed to identify a reduced risk of second stroke or death, even though the treatment reduces risk in reality. This erroneous outcome is best described as

A. observe bias.

B. selection bias.

C. confounding bias.

D. type I error.

E. type II error.

FURTHER READING

Chan AW, Tetzlaff JM, Gøtzsche PC, et al. SPIRIT 2013 explanation and elaboration: guidance for protocols of clinical trials. *BMJ*. 2013; 346.

Lambert J. Statistics in brief: how to assess bias in clinical studies? *Clin Orthop Relat Res*. 2011; 469(6):1794-1796.

Little RJ, D'Agostino R, Cohen ML, et al. The prevention and treatment of missing data in clinical trials. *N Engl J Med*. 2012; 367:1355-1360.

Schulz KF, Altman DG, Moher D; CONSORT Group. CONSORT 2010 statement: updated guidelines for reporting parallel group randomized trials. *Ann Intern Med*. 2010; 152(11):726-732.

Senn S. Seven myths of randomisation in clinical trials. *Stat Med*. 2013; 32(9):1439-1450.

Pocock SJ, Assmann SE, Enos LE, Kasten LE. Subgroup analysis, covariate adjustment and baseline comparisons in clinical trial reporting: current practice and problems. *Stat Med*. 2002; 21(19):2917-2930.

Zarin DA, Tse T, Williams RJ, Califf RM, Ide NC. The ClinicalTrials.gov results database—update and key issues. *N Engl J Med*. 2011; 364:852-860.

Web Resources

1. ClinicalTrials.gov
2. Cochrane Library. http://www.cochrane.org.
3. Consort Guidelines. http://www.consort-statement.org.
4. International Conference on Harmonization. http://www.ich.org.

REFERENCES

Introduction

Woosley RL, Cossman J. Drug development and the FDA's Critical Path Initiative. *Clin Pharmacol Ther*. 2007; 81(1):129-133.

Clinical Trials Design

Tunis SR, Stryer DB, Clancy CM. Practical clinical trials increasing value of clinical research for decision making in clinical and health policy. *JAMA*. 2003; 2 90(12):1624-1632.

Phase I Clinical Trials

Collins JM. Innovations in phase 1 trial design: where do we go next? *Clin Cancer Res*. 2000;6(10):3801-3802.

Conclusions and Limitations

Sung NS, Crowley WF Jr, Genel M, et al. Central challenges facing the national clinical research enterprise. *JAMA*. 2003; 289(10), 1278-1287.

8

Diagnostic Testing

Clinicians need making diagnoses for symptoms or abnormalities presented by their patients with tests. Meanwhile, new diagnostic tests are developed rapidly and existing tests are continuously being improved. In addition, the clinician needs to know which patients are likely to benefit from testing, the likelihood that a patient with a positive test actually has the disease, and the likelihood that a patient with a negative test does not have the disease. A competent clinician can use good judgment, a thorough knowledge of the literature and somewhat intuitive approach to this information. However, there are basic principles the clinician should understand about the evaluating and interpreting diagnostic tests.

A **diagnostic test** is a test performed in a laboratory, such as a histopathological examination or microbiological culture; it applies equally to other clinical information such as history, physical examination, and imaging procedures. A series of combined findings may also serve as a diagnostic test.

Diagnostic tests may be used to diagnose primary disease that is to identify the disease for the first time in a patient and identify disease subtypes such as hemorrhagic stroke or ischemic stroke; to predict treatment response, that is to test characteristics of patients or their diseases that may identify the type of treatment to maximize the chances of a favorable response; to detect residual disease, such as to identify cancer cells or infectious agents that remain after treatment is completed; to predict prognosis, a test result may indicate the likely course of disease and the probability of cure; monitor remission or progression, if a disease is in remission, testing may help

detect the return or progression of disease; screen, for example, serum antibodies, skin test reactions, imaging results, cytological findings, etc., may point towards the presence of disease before signs or symptoms become manifested.

DESIGN OF STUDIES TO EVALUATE TEST PERFORMANCE

There are different requirements for the evaluation of diagnostic tests in different situations. Both new and existing tests, like therapeutic procedures, need to be studied, evaluated, and selected based on rigorous empirical data prior to incorporating them into clinical practice. In studying diagnostic tests, comparing the results of the test with that of a **"gold standard"** in both patient (diseased) and control (not diseased) groups is the key to evaluating performance.

GOLD STANDARD

"Gold standard", that are generally accepted as the best available indication of the true presence or absence of disease. The assessment of a test's accuracy rests on knowledge of whether the disease is truly present or not. One often cannot know disease status with absolute certainty. However, for almost all conditions there are findings referred to as gold standard. The gold standard may be the results of a biopsy, surgical confirmation, autopsy, or other definitive tests. In practice, the gold standard is often elusive. Sometimes the standard of accuracy is itself a relatively simple and inexpensive test. More often, one must turn to relatively elaborate, expensive, or risky tests to be certain whether the disease is present or absent.

At least initially, clinician and patients prefer a simpler test, since using more accurate ways of establishing the truth is almost always more costly and more dangerous. For example, chest x-rays and sputum smears are used to determine the nature of pneumonia, rather than lung biopsy with examination of the diseased lung tissue. Similarly, electrocardiography and serum enzyme assays are often used to establish the diagnosis of acute myocardial infarction, rather than catheterization.

In practice, sometimes it is impossible for physicians to find information on how well the tests they use comparing with a thoroughly trustworthy standard, because no such standard exists. They have to choose another test as their standard of validity that admittedly is imperfect but is considered the best one that is available. This may force physicians to compare one weak test against another, with one test being accepted as a standard of validity because it has had longer use or is considered superior by a consensus of experts. In this way, a paradox may arise, for if a new test is compared with an old but inaccurate standard test, the new test may seem worse when it is actually better. For example, if the new test is better at detecting cases than the standard test, some diseased patients identified by the new test as positive would be considered false positives in relation to the old test.

The results of follow-up also can serve as gold standards for diseases that are not self-limited and ordinarily become overt in a matter of a few months or years after they are first suspected. Most chronic degenerative diseases including cancers fall into this category. For them, validation is possible with the results of follow up even if on the spot confirmation of a test's performance is not feasible because the immediately available gold standard is too inaccurate, risky, involved, or expensive. The length of the follow-up period must be long enough for the disease to manifest.

STUDY SUBJECTS

The group of study patients should mirror the spec-trum of disease found in the types of patients that would be tested in clinical practice to help ensure that the research results can be extrapolated to general clinical practice. Initial reports describing a new test may include only patients with obvious and overt manifestations of disease and thus end up excluding the milder cases (the shades of gray) who are more likely to have false negative tests. Likewise, people in whom disease is only suspected may have other conditions that cause a positive test, thereby increasing the false-positive rate. Early research designs evaluating tests often contrast a test's results in people who are clearly diseased (e.g., hospitalized patients with advanced disease) with results obtained in people who are clearly not diseased (e.g., medical student volunteers), and the resulting black-versus-white comparisons provide an overly optimistic picture of the test's performance among the type of patients typically encountered in real practice situations.

Measures of test performance, such as sensitivity and specificity [described below], may represent average values for a population. Unless the condition for which a test is to be used is narrowly defined, the indices may vary in different medical subgroups. For successful use of a test, separate indices of accuracy may be needed for pertinent individual subgroups within the spectrum of tested patients. This standard is met when results for indices of accuracy are reported for a range of demographic or clinical subgroups.

SAMPLE SIZE

When designing diagnostic test studies, sample size calculations should be performed in order to guarantee that study findings are sufficiently precise to be relied upon for purposes of setting policy and guiding practice. Too small a sample size may miss a significant effect when one exists. But too large a sample size will entail unnecessary costs and may establish a statistical significance that is clinically irrelevant. In determining the desired sample size, for the study the investigator must specify how precisely these measures are to be estimated. For sensitivity and specificity, the standard formula for a binomial proportion is used:

$$n = (\frac{u_\alpha}{\delta})^2 p(1-p)$$

Where n is the number of abnormal (diseased) or normal (healthy) subjects to be included in the study, δ is admissible error, P is the estimated sensitivity (or specificity) for the test, u_α is the u value for the cumulative probability equal to α/2. This formula is suitable when the estimated sensitivity or specificity is around 50%. When the estimated sensitivity (or specificity) is ⩽20% or ⩾80% the corrected formula is:

$$n = [57.3u_\alpha/\sin^{-1}(\delta/\sqrt{p(1-p)})]^2$$

BLIND TO ASSESS THE RESULTS

Blinding is important to judging the results of studies evaluating the performance of a diagnostic test. Those who perform the test must be unaware of the true diagnosis to avoid bias. In studies to evaluate the reproducibility of a measurement technique the observers must be unaware the results of their previous measurement(s) on the same individual.

DETERMINATION OF THE CUTOFF VALUE

The goal of evaluating diagnostic test performance is to determine how well the test discriminates between those who are diseased and those who are not diseased. For almost all tests the distributions of results for these two groups overlaps to some extent, so a cutoff score must be established to discriminate best between diseased and not diseased persons. When a new diagnostic test is developed or when a diagnostic test is to be used in a clinical condition different from the one for which the test was developed, the test's cutoff score may require (re-)determination. This determination or re-determination may be based on biological, clinical or demographic situations, but statistical methods are also useful. Analytical and empirical approaches for defining reliable and valid cutoff points are described in section below on "The cutoff value of diagnostic test."

DATA ANALYSIS OF DIAGNOSTIC TESTING

In a perfect situation, medical diagnostic tests would give absolute correct results. For example, patient could undergo a diagnostic test that would unequivocally determine whether lung cancer was present. A positive test result would indicate that cancer was present and a negative test result would indicate that cancer was absent. In reality, however, every test is fallible.

When evaluating the performance of a diagnostic test, the first step is to determine the true status of subjects or patients according to the gold standard. Then, the same study subjects are tested by the diagnostic test being evaluated. Consider a gold standard and diagnostic test that have only positive or negative results (Table 8-1). After the two tests are performed, one of four possible scenarios will occur. The "true" disease status is determined by the most definitive diagnostic method, which is gold standard. In cell a, the disease of interest is present and the test result is positive, is a "true positive" result. In cell d, the disease is absent and the test result is negative, is a "true-negative" result. In both of these cells, the test result agrees with the actual status of the disease. Cell b represents individuals without the disease who have a positive test result. Since these test results incorrectly suggest that the disease is present, they are considered to be "false-positives". Individuals in cell c have the disease but have negative test results. These results are designated "false-negatives" because they incorrectly suggest that the disease is absent.

Table 8-1 Analysis the Results of New Diagnostic Test and Gold Standard

New diagnostic test	Gold standard Disease present	Disease absent	Total
Positive	True positive (a)	False positive (b)	a+b
Negative	False Negative (c)	True Negative (d)	c+d
Total	a+c	b+d	N

ACCURACY OF DIAGNOSTIC TEST

Accuracy refers to the concordance between the results of the diagnostic test and gold standard. Accuracy is also call validity, which is a crucial indicator of the quality and usefulness of a test and can be expressed through sensitivity and specificity, positive and negative diagnostic likelihood ratios, etc. Each measure of accuracy should be used in combination with its complementary measure.

Sensitivity and Specificity

Sensitivity and specificity are terms used to describe the validity of the new test relative to the gold standard.

Sensitivity: Sensitivity is the ability of tests to detect disease when it is present and is defined as the percentage of persons with the disease of interest who have positive test results (Table 7-1). It is a measure of the probability of correctly detecting a condition and is calculated as follows:

$$\text{Sensitivity} = \frac{\text{True-positives}}{\text{True-positives} + \text{False-negatives}} = \frac{a}{a+c}$$

If a test is negative in a patient with disease, it is a false-negative result. The false-negative rate is the proportion of those with disease ($a+c$) who erroneously test negative(c). The sensitivity (true-positive rate) and the false-negative rate are complementary and add to 1.

The greater the sensitivity of a test, the more likely it is that the test will detect persons who have the disease of interest. Tests with greater sensitivity are useful clinically to rule out the presence of a disease. That is, a negative result for a highly sensitive test virtually excludes the possibility that the patient has the disease.

We use the validity of serum creatine kinase for diagnosis of acute myocardial infarction, using coronary angiography as the gold standard as example to illustrate the accuracy, the data are listed in Table 8-2.

Table 8-2 Accuracy of Serum Creatine Kinase

| serum creatine kinase | Acute myocardial infarction | | Total |
	yes	no	
≥80 u/L(postive)	226	24	250
<80 u/L(negative)	24	121	145
Total	250	145	395

We can see that both serum creatine kinase and coronary angiography identify 250 cases as having an acute myocardial infarction. However, the table shows that the persons identified by these two methods are not entirely the same. Among the 250 cases of acute myocardial infarction identified with coronary angiography (the gold standard), 226 tested positive by serum creatine kinase (true positive), and 24 cases tested negative (false negative); among the 145 cases without acute myocardial infarction as determined by the gold standard of angiography, 121 cases tested negative with serum creatine kinase (true negative), and 24 cases tested positive (false positive). Therefore, the different indicators of validity of serum creatine kinase are calculated as follows:

$$\text{Sensitivity} = \frac{226}{250} \times 100\% = 90.40\%$$

$$\text{False negative rate (misdiagnosed)} = \frac{24}{250} \times 100\%$$
$$= 9.96\%$$

Specificity: Specificity is the ability of a test to exclude disease when it is absent. Specificity of a test is defined as the percentage of persons without the disease of interest who have negative test results. Specificity is calculated as follows:

$$\text{Specificity} = \frac{\text{True-negatives}}{\text{True-negatives} + \text{False-positives}} = \frac{d}{b+d}$$

Among those free of disease, there are true negatives and false positives. The false-positive rate is the proportion of those without disease ($b+d$) in whom test results are incorrectly positive (b). The specificity (true-negative rate) and the false-positive rate are complementary and add to 1.

The greater the specificity of a test, the more likely it is that persons without the disease of interest will be excluded from consideration of having the disease. Very specific tests often are used to confirm the presence of a disease. If the test is highly specific, a positive test result would strongly suggest the presence of the disease of interest.

In general, the reported results of sensitivity and specificity in the literature may represent the average values for a wide range of populations. Unless the conditions or circumstances in which a test is to be used are narrowly defined, the indices may vary in different practice situations. Separate indices of accuracy may be needed for pertinent individual sub-groups within the spectrum of tested patients.

The specificity and false positive rate of above example is as:

$$\text{Specificity (true negative rate)} = \frac{121}{145} \times 100\% = 83.45\%$$

$$\text{False positive rate (misdiagnosed)} = \frac{24}{145} \times 100\%$$
$$= 16.55\%$$

Likelihood Ratios

The Likelihood Ratio (LR) is the probability of a particular test result for a person with the disease of interest divided by the probability of that test result for a person without the disease of interest. Therefore, LRs are defined for either positive or negative test results.

Positive likelihood ratios: The likelihood ratio for a positive test result (LR+) is the probability of a positive test result for a person with the disease of interest divided by the probability of a positive test result for a person without the disease. Mathematically, the LR+ is calculated as

LR+=sensitivity/(1−specificity)

An LR+ with a value of one indicates a test with no value in sorting out persons with and without the disease of interest, as the probability of a positive test result is equally likely among persons affected and unaffected with the disease of interest. The smallest possible value of the LR+ occurs when the numerator is minimized (sensitivity=0), producing an LR+ of zero. The maximum value of the LR+ occurs when the denominator is minimized (specificity=1, so 1−specificity= 0), resulting in an LR+ of positive infinity. Values of the LR+ greater than one correspond to situations in which persons affected with the disease of interest are more likely to have a positive test result than unaffected persons. The larger the value of the LR+, the stronger the association are between having a positive test result and having the disease of interest.

A diagnostic test with a large LR+ value increases the suspicion of disease for patients with positive test results. The larger the size of the LR+ is, the better

the diagnostic value of the test is. On somewhat arbitrary grounds, an LR+ value of 10 or greater is often perceived as an indication of a test of high diagnostic value.

Negative likelihood ratio: Similar reasoning applies to the LR−, except in the opposite direction. An LR−with a value of one indicates a test with no value in sorting out persons with and without the disease of interest, as the probability of a negative test result is equally likely among persons affected and unaffected with the disease of interest

LR−= (1−sensitivity)/specificity

The smallest value of the LR-occurs when the numerator is minimized (sensitivity=1, so 1−sensitivity=0), resulting in an LR-of zero. The largest value of the LR−occurs when the denominator is minimized (specificity=0), resulting in an LR−of positive infinity. A diagnostic test with a small LR−value decreases the suspicion of disease for patients with negative test results. The smaller the size of the LR−is, the better the diagnostic value of the test is. Again on somewhat arbitrary grounds, an LR−value of 0.1 or less is often perceived as an indication of a test of high diagnostic value.

The LRs in above example is:

$$LR+ = \frac{226/250}{24/145} \times 100\% = 5.45$$

$$LR- = \frac{25/250}{121/145} \times 100\% = 0.12$$

Youden Index

Youden Index (YI) can be defined as:
$$YI = Se + Sp - 1$$

It ranges between 0 and 1. Complete separation of the distributions of the marker values for the diseased and healthy populations results in YI=1 whereas complete overlap gives YI=0. The Youden Index is used to denote the overall performance of a test and provides a criterion for choosing the "optimal" threshold value. YI is also frequently used in practice. YI in the above example is 0.90+0.83−1=0.73.

Agreement rate

Agreement rate also called "accuracy rate". It is

the agreement between the results of diagnostic test and gold standard. It is the number and proportion of all the observations which have been classified correctly by the test.

$$\text{Agreement rate} = \frac{a+d}{N} \times 100\%$$

$$\text{Agreement rate in the above example} = \frac{226+121}{395}$$

$$\times 100\% = 87.85\%.$$

RELIABILITY OF DIAGNOSTIC TEST

Reliability, or **reproducibility**, is the ability of a test to yield consistent results when repeated on the same patient or specimen at different times or in different circumstances. A test with perfect reproducibility should give the same result when repeated on the same sample or patient. However, there almost always are sources of variation in test results that relate to biological variability in the phenomenon being measured (within person variability), in the interpretation of a single observer (intra-rater reliability), or the interpretation among different observers (inter-observer reliability), or in the mechanical performance of the test itself in one or more laboratories (intra-and inter-laboratory variability). These sources of variation may be both random and non-random.

Assessment of reproducibility needs comparing the results of repeated applications or interpretations of the same test, allowing estimation of coefficients of "agreement," such as Cohen's kappa or the intraclass correlation coefficient.

Cohen's Kappa

Cohen's Kappa is a measure of agreement between two tests or repeated tests between different times or different circumstances. The calculation of Cohen's Kappa is as the following formula:

$$kappa = \frac{\text{(observed agreement\%)} - \text{(agreement expected by chance\%)}}{100\% - \text{(agreement expected by chance\%)}}$$

The calculation of Cohen's kappa is illustrated by the 2 by 2 table for results obtained from two pathologists' laboratories (Table 8-3).

Table 8-3 Kappa Analysis between Two Pathologist on 68 Specimens

Pathologist B	Pathologist A		Total by B
	+	–	
+	a (36)	b (2)	$a+b$ (r_1 38)
–	c (4)	d (26)	$c+d$ (r_2 30)
Total by A	$a+c$ (c_1 40)	$b+d$ (c_2 28)	$a+b+c+d$ (n 68)

$$\text{observed agreement } (P_0) = \frac{a+d}{N} \times 100\% = \frac{36+26}{68}$$

$$\times 100\% = 91.18\%$$

$$\text{agreement of chance } (P_c) = \frac{r_1 c_1/N + r_2 c_2/N}{N} \times 100\%$$

$$= \frac{(38\times40)/68 + (30\times28)/68}{68} \times 100\% = 51.04\%$$

$$\text{potential agreement beyond chance} = 1 - P_c = 1 - 0.5104$$
$$= 0.4896 \text{(or)} 48.96\%$$

$$\text{actual agreement beyond chance} = p_0 - p_c = 0.9118 - 0.5104$$
$$= 0.4014 \text{(or } 40.14\%)$$

$$Kappa = \frac{\text{actual agreement beyond chance}}{1 - \text{agreement of chance}}$$

$$= \frac{P_o - P_c}{1 - P_c} = \frac{0.4014}{0.4896} = 0.8199 \text{(or } 81.99\%)$$

Kappa ranges between−1 and +1, and indicates the level of agreement beyond chance when two tests (or observers) are classifying the same set of specimens into two or more exclusive categories (e.g., infected/not infected or normal/mild/moderate/severe/critical). A kappa of 0 indicates no agreement beyond that expected by chance, 1 indicates complete agreement, and−1 indicates a inverse (or contrary) agreement. When the classification categories are ordered and more than three (e.g., normal/mild/ severe/critical), Cohen's Kappa tends to underestimates the degree of actual agreement, and a weighted Kappa or other statistic is preferable. Kappa values for components of the clinical examination often range between 0.4 and 0.7, which indicates the source of many differences among clinicians.

Intra-Rater Agreement

This is a measure of the level of agreement beyond

chance, typically quantified by Cohen's Kappa, that a test or observer has with itself ("intra" = within) when repeated on the same set of materials. For example, it could measure the degree to which radiologists provide the same diagnosis when they re-read the same film without knowledge of their earlier diagnosis.

Inter-Rater Agreement

This measures the level of agreement beyond chance, typically quantified by Cohen's Kappa, for two different tests or observers ("inter" = between) when performed on the same materials. For example, it could measure how well the diagnoses of two different radiologists agree when reading the same films.

EFFECTIVE OF A DIAGNOSTIC TEST

Sensitivity and specificity are descriptors of the accuracy of a test itself. While test is used in clinical practice, two measures concerning the estimation of the probability of the presence or absence of disease are the **positive predictive value** (PPV) and the **negative predictive value** (NPV).

Positive Predictive Value

The PPV is defined as the percentage of persons with positive test results who actually have the disease of interest. The PPV therefore, allows us to estimate how likely it is that the disease of interest is present when the test is positive. Referring again to Table 8-1, the PPV is calculated as follows:

$$PPV = \frac{\text{True-positives}}{\text{True-positives+False-positives}} = \frac{a}{a+b}$$

The calculation of the PPV for the serum creatine kinase test described in Table 8-2 is

$$PPV = \frac{\text{True-positives}}{\text{True-positives+False-positives}} = \frac{a}{a+b}$$

$$= \frac{226}{226+24} = \frac{226}{250} = 0.904$$

The average probability of acute myocardial infarction in this sample prior to serum creatine

kinase test was 226 affected subjects of 395 total subjects, or 57%. After the serum creatine kinase test, the probability of acute myocardial infarction for a subject who with a positive test result increased to 88%.

Negative Predictive Value

The NPV is the percentage of persons with negative test results who do not have the disease of interest.

$$NPV = \frac{\text{True-negatives}}{\text{True-negatives+False-negatives}} = \frac{d}{c+d}$$

The NPV for the serum creatine kinase test $= \frac{121}{121+24}$

$$= 0.83$$

Sensitivity and specificity are characteristics of a screening or diagnostic test itself. In contrast, the predictive value of a test is not a property of the test alone. It is determined by the prevalence of disease in the population being tested, as well as by the sensitivity and specificity of the test. Here prevalence has its customary meaning---the proportion of persons in a defined population at a given point in time with the condition in question. Prevalence is also a "prior probability", or the probability of disease before the test result is known.

Factors affecting predictive value

It is important to appreciate that the usefulness of a test changes as the clinical situation changes. Specifically, the pretest probability of the presence of disease in an individual, or the prevalence of disease in a population, greatly influences the predictive value.

The mathematical formula relating sensitivity, specificity, and prevalence to positive predictive value is derived from Bayes's theorem of conditional probabilities:

$$PPV = \frac{\text{sensitivity} \times \text{prevalence}}{\text{sensitivity} \times \text{prevalence} + (1-\text{specificity}) \times (1-\text{prevalence})}$$

$$NPV = \frac{\text{specificity} \times (1-\text{prevalence})}{(1-\text{sensitivity}) \times \text{prevalence} + \text{specificity}(1-\text{prevalence})}$$

The more sensitive a test is, the higher will be its

negative predictive value (the more confident the clinician can be that a negative test result rules out the disease being sought). Conversely, the more specific the test is, the higher will be its positive predictive value (the more confident the clinician can be that a positive test confirms or rules in the diagnosis being sought). Because predictive value is also influenced by prevalence, it is not independent of the setting in which the test is used. Positive results for a very specific diagnostic test (with very high specificity), when applied to patients with a low likelihood of having the disease, will be largely false positives. Similarly, negative results, even for a very sensitive test, when applied to patients with a high chance of having the disease, are likely to be false negatives. In sum, the interpretation of a positive or negative diagnostic test result varies from setting to setting according to the prevalence of disease in the particular setting (Table 8-4).

It may not be intuitively obvious what prevalence has to do with an individual patient. For those who are skeptical, it might help to consider how a test would perform at the extremes of prevalence. Remember that no matter how sensitive and specific a test might be, there will be a small proportion of patients who are misclassified by it. Imagine a population in which no one has the disease. In such a group all positive results, even for a very specific test, will be false positives. Therefore, as the prevalence of disease in a population approaches zero, the positive predictive value of a test also approaches zero. As prevalence approaches 100%, negative predictive value approaches zero.

When the prevalence of disease in the population tested is relatively high, the test performs well at identifying those who truly are diseased. But at a lower prevalence, the positive predictive value drops to nearly zero, and the test is virtually useless for diagnosing disease. As sensitivity and specificity fall, the influence of changes in prevalence on predictive value becomes more acute.

Diagnostic and Treatment Yield

Tests with high sensitivity and specificity have fewer false positive or false negative results and lead to more people receiving appropriate diagnoses (diagnostic yield) and appropriate treatment (therapeutic yield). For example, the enhanced accuracy of fluorescence cystoscopy compared with white light cystoscopy alone for detecting recurrence of bladder carcinoma in situ has led to a substantial increase in lesions being identified and treated at initial diagnosis and a significantly reduced rate of recurrence.

THE CUTOFF VALUE OF DIAGNOSTIC TEST

CONSIDERATIONS IN CHOOSING A CUTOFF VALUE

In some situations, a test result can have only one of two possible results; positive or negative. In other circumstance, multiple levels of values, or a continuous range of values, can occur, and one must choose

Table 8-4 The Relationship between Prevalence, Sensitivity, Specificity and Predictive value

Prevalence (%)	Sensitivity (%)	Specificity (%)	Test	Gold standard		Total	PPV (%)	NPV (%)
				Diabetes	Normal			
1.5	22.9	99.8	+	34	20	54	63.0	
			−	116	9830	9946		98.8
			Total	150	9850	10000		
1.5	44.3	99.0	+	66	98	164	40.2	
			−	84	9752	9836		99.1
			Total	150	9850	10000		
2.5	44.3	99.0	+	111	97	208	53.3	
			−	139	9653	9792		98.6
			Total	250	9750	10000		

a cut-off point on the continuum between normal and abnormal. A test that is both highly sensitivity and highly specificity is desirable in theory but is often unobtainable in practice. Instead, one characteristic (e.g., sensitivity) can be increased, but only at the expense of the other (e.g., specificity). Table 8-5 demonstrates this interrelationship for the diagnosis of diabetes. If we require that a Hemoglobin A1c (HbA1c) be greater than 7.7% to diagnose diabetes, almost all of the people diagnosed as "diabetic" would certainly have the disease, but many other people with diabetes would be missed using this definition. The test would be very specific at the expense of sensitivity. At the other extreme, if anyone with a HbA1c of greater than 5.1% were diagnosed as diabetic, very few people with the disease would be missed, but most normal people would be falsely labeled as having diabetes. The test would then be sensitive but nonspecific. There is no way, using a single HbA1c determination under standard conditions, that one can improve both the sensitivity and specificity of the test at the same time.

When making decisions about the optimal cutoff value, the test characteristics, the consequences of diagnostic mistakes, the costs of testing and treatment, and the effectiveness of treatment should be taken into account. Thus, with a test for a disease that is likely to be fatal or have serious disabling consequences if not identified accurately, and for which there is an effective therapy, higher sensitivity will be favored. However, for a disease in which a delayed diagnosis would not have serious consequences and the costs of evaluating patients with false positive tests would be high, a higher specificity would be favored. When both false positive and false nega-tive results are deemed to be equally important, the cutoff value can be selected as the crossover point of the frequency distributions of the results for diseased patients and the normal population, but statistical methods for choosing the cutoff are generally preferable.

DETERMINING TEST CUTOFF VALUE

Statistical Methods

A. Mean ± 2SD Method: When the test measure in question appears to have a normal distribution, the mean ± 2SD define the 95% confidence interval of the distribution. Therefore one can (arbitrarily) define the value that falls in the extreme top or bottom 2.5% of the distribution as abnormally high or low, respectively.

B. Percentile Method: When the test measure does not appear as a normal distribution, one can specify the cutoff (arbitrarily) according to the top and/or bottom percentile of the distribution.

C. ROC Method: For diagnostic tests that produce results on a continuous scale of measurement, an **ROC (receiver operator characteristic curve)** can be constructed by plotting the true-positive rate (sensitivity) against the false-positive rate (1-specificity) over a range of test values. This curve derives its name from its first application—measuring the ability of radar operators to distinguish radar signals from noise. The values on the axes run from a probability of 0 to 1.0 (or, alternatively, from 0 to 100%). The ROC is thus a graphic way to express the relationship between sensitivity and specificity. Tests that discriminate well crowd toward the upper left corner of the ROC curve; for them, as the sensitivity is

Table 8-5   Trade-off between Sensitivity and Specificity when Diagnosing Diabetes

HbA1c (%)	Sensitivity (%)	Specificity (%)	HbA1c (%)	Sensitivity (%)	Specificity (%)
5.1	99.7	9.8	6.5 *	81.1	83.3
5.3	99.2	19.1	6.7	74.8	89.0
5.5	98.3	31.4	6.9	68.7	92.4
5.7	96.6	43.8	7.1	62.8	95.2
5.9	94.3	54.3	7.3	57.4	97.4
6.1	90.6	66.9	7.5	51.1	98.2
6.3	86.1	76.3	7.7	46.4	98.6

progressively increased (the cutoff point is lowered) there is little or no loss in specificity. The area under the ROC curve serves as an overall measure of test performance, with an area of 1 indicating a perfect test and an area of 0.5 indicating a test that is unable to distinguish persons with and without the disease of interest (Figure 8-1).

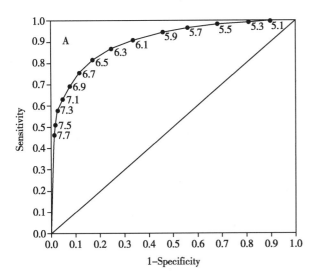

Figure 8-1 The ROC of HbA1c to diagnose diabetes

The respective areas under the ROC curves for two (or more) diagnostic tests for a particular disease can be used to identify the test that will provide the greater diagnostic value. ROC curves also can be used to comparing the performance of different observers (Figure 8-2).

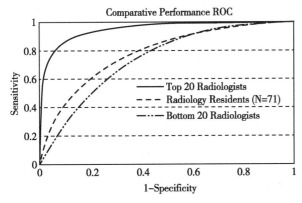

Figure 8-2 ROC Curve for comparing the performance of different kinds of radiologist

Clinical Considerations

The cutoff value for a test can also be decided based on the known impact of the measure as a risk factor

for disease. For example, defining the normal cholesterol as lower than 6.5mmol/L helps to identify individuals who are at increased risk of atherosclerotic heart disease may benefit from cholesterol lowing strategies. Sometimes the cutoff value is determined based on the prognostic importance of the measurement for a particular disease. For example, among patients infected with Human Immunodeficiency Virus (HIV), a CD4$^+$ cell count of less than 400/ml identifies individuals who are highly likely to develop serious infections unless treated with antiretroviral therapy.

IMPROVE THE EFFICIENCY OF DIAGNOSTIC TEST

Different diagnostic tests are usually sensitive to different aspects of the disease. Combining multiple diagnostic tests may thus serve as a composite diagnostic test process with higher sensitivity and specificity that detects the presence of the disease more accurately.

MULTIPLE TESTS

When multiple tests are performed, and all are positive or all are negative, the interpretation is straightforward. All too often, however, some test results are positive and others are negative, and interpretation becomes more complicated. In this section, we discuss the principles by which multiple tests are applied and interpreted. Multiple tests can be applied in two general ways. They can be used in parallel, and a positive result of any test is considered evidence for disease. Or they can be done serially (i.e., consecutively), based on the results of the previous test. For serial testing, all tests must give a positive result for the diagnosis to be made, because the diagnostic process is stopped when a negative result is obtained.

Parallel tests

Multiple tests done in parallel generally can increase sensitivity and the negative predictive value for a disease above that of the individual tests. On the other hand, specificity and positive predictive value are lowered. Thus, disease is less likely to be missed, but more false-positive diagnoses are likely to be seen. The degree to which sensitivity and negative predictive value increase depends on the extent to which the tests identify disease that is missed by the other tests used. For example, if two tests are used in parallel with 60% and 80% sensitivities, the sensitivity of the parallel testing will be only 80% if the better test identifies all the cases found by the less sensitive test. If the two tests each detect all the cases missed by the other, the sensitivity of **parallel test** is, of course, 100%. If the two test results are completely independent of each other, then the sensitivity of the parallel testing will be 92% based on the following formula:

The sensitivity of the parallel testing =

(Sensitivity of test A) + (Sensitivity of test B) × (1-Sensitivity of test A)

The specificity of the parallel testing = (The specificity of test A) × (The specificity of test B)

Parallel testing is particularly useful when the clinician is faced with the need for a very sensitive test but has available only two or more relatively insensitive tests that measure different clinical phenomena. By using the tests in parallel, the net effect is a more sensitive diagnostic strategy.

Serial tests

Physicians most commonly use serial testing strategies in clinical situations where rapid assessment of patients is not required, such as in office practices and hospital clinics where ambulatory patients are followed over time. Serial testing is also used when some of the tests are expensive or risky; these tests are employed only after simpler and safer tests suggest the presence of disease. **Serial test** leads to less laboratory use than parallel testing, because additional evaluation is contingent on prior test results. However, serial testing takes more time because additional tests are ordered only after the results of previous ones become available.

Serial testing maximizes specificity and positive predictive value but lowers sensitivity and negative predictive value. One ends up more confident that a positive test result represents true disease but runs an increased risk that disease will be missed. Serial testing is particularly useful when none of the individual tests available to a clinician is highly specific. If two test results are completely independent of each other, then the sensitivity and specificity of the serial testing will be calculated according to the following formula:

The sensitivity of the series testing = (The sensitivity of test A) × (The sensitivity of test B)

The specificity of the series testing = (The specificity of test A) + (The specificity of test B) (1-The specificity of test A)

In practice, however, it is rarely the case that the performance of two (or more) diagnostic tests is completely independent when they are applied for diagnosing a disease.

The pattern of diagnostic results obtained by parallel and series testing using two tests is shown in Table 8-6, and Table 8-7 provides a hypothetical example of the results of using two diagnostic tests for diabetes, urine sugar and blood sugar, employed sequentially and in parallel.

Table 8-6 Results of Multiple Testing Strategies

Test A	Test B	Parallel test	Serial test
+	+	+	+
+	−	+	−
−	+	+	−
−	−	−	−

Table 8-7 Urine and Blood Sugar Tests for Diabetes Used in Parallel or Serially

Diagnostic test			
Urine sugar	Blood sugar	Diabetes	Non-diabetes
+	−	14	10
−	+	33	11
+	+	117	21
−	−	35	7599
Total		199	7641

Blood sugar test:

$$\text{Sensitivity} = \frac{33+117}{199} \times 100\% = 75.38\%$$

$$\text{Specificity} = \frac{10+7599}{7641} \times 100\% = 99.58\%$$

Urine sugar test:

$$\text{Sensitivity} = \frac{14+117}{199} \times 100\% = 65.83\%$$

$$\text{Specificity} = \frac{11+7599}{7641} \times 100\% = 99.59\%$$

Series test:

$$\text{Sensitivity} = \frac{117}{199} \times 100\% = 58.79\%$$

$$\text{Specificity} = \frac{10+11+7599}{7641} \times 100\% = 99.73\%$$

Parallel test:

$$\text{Sensitivity} = \frac{14+33+117}{199} \times 100\% = 82.41\%$$

$$\text{Specificity} = \frac{7599}{7641} \times 100\% = 99.45\%$$

SELECTING HIGH RISK POPULATIONS

In practice, diagnostic tests are most helpful when the presence of disease neither very likely nor very unlikely. When disease is highly unlikely, one can increase the yield of a test by selecting a population for testing that has a higher prevalence of disease. There are a variety of ways in which the probability of a disease can be increased before using a diagnostic test.

Referral process

The referral process is one of the most common ways in which the probability of disease is increased. Referral to a teaching hospital or other specialty hospital increases the chance that significant disease underlies patients' complaints. Therefore, relatively more aggressive use of diagnostic tests might be justified in these settings. In primary care practice, on the other hand, and particularly among patients without complaints, the chance of finding disease is considerable smaller, and tests should be used more sparingly.

Selected demographic groups

In a given setting, doctors can increase the yield of diagnostic tests by applying them to demographic groups known to be at higher risk for a disease. For example, a man of 65 is 15 times more likely to have coronary artery disease as the cause of atypical chest pain than a woman of 30.

Specifics of the clinical situation

The presence or absence of symptoms, signs, and disease risk factors all raise or lower the probability of finding a disease and exert the strongest influence on the decision of when to order tests. For example, a woman with chest pain is more likely to have coronary disease if she has typical angina and hypertension and she smokes. In contrast, a negative exercise stress test in an asymptomatic 35 year old man merely confirms the already low probability of coronary artery disease.

Because prevalence of disease is such a powerful determinant of the usefulness of a diagnostic test, clinicians must consider the probability of disease before ordering a test. However until recently, clinicians could only rely on clinical observations and their experience to estimate the pretest probability of a disease. Now, however, research using large clinical computer data bases can provide quantitative estimates of the probability of disease for various combinations of clinical findings. Using these kinds of data can lead to more accurate and effective diagnostic testing.

SCREENIG

In medicine, **screening** is used in a population to identify the possible presence of an as-yet-undiagnosed disease in individuals without signs or symptoms.Figure 8-3 is a schematic representation of the course of disease over time, and illustrates the possibility of detecting the presence of disease earlier using a screening test, thereby allowing for more effective treatment and prolonged survival. The criteria for successful screening program is listed in

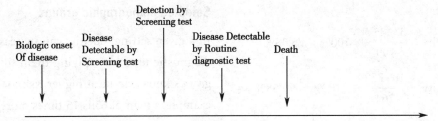

Figure 8-3 The natural history of a disease over time

Table 8-8.Inherent in this schematic diagram are two important concepts: (1) a screening test can identify individuals with a disease before the presence of a disease is detected by routine diagnosis (eg, when symptoms occur), and (2) treatment at the time of detection by screening, as opposed to the time of routine diagnosis, results in an improved chance of survival.

It has long been known that length of survival from time of diagnosis of a disease related to the stage of this disease. For example, researchers postulated that by screening asymptomatic women with mammography, breast cancer could be detected at an earlier stage, and, therefore, affected women as a group would experience increased survival. This logic seems infallible, but two important biases—**lead-time bias** and **length-biased sampling**—must be considered when evaluating any screening program.

As illustrated in Figure 8-4, lead-time bias is an increase in survival as measured from detection of disease to death, without lengthening of life. Note in Figure 8-4 that the person detected with screen-

ing and the person detected without screening die at exactly the same time, but the time from diagnosis until death is greater for the screened patient because the cancer was recognized at an earlier point in time. The time from early diagnosis by screening to routine diagnosis is defined as the lead time.

Length-biased sampling occurs when disease detected by a screening program is less aggressive than disease detected without screening. On average, breast cancers detected by a screening program may be less aggressive than cancers that are diagnosed when symptoms appear. This occurs because less aggressive cancers typically grow at a slower pace than more aggressive malignancies, and therefore the length of time that a cancer is detectable by screening is greater for slow-growing neoplasms. If length of survival is measured, individuals with breast cancers detected by screening appear to live longer, in part because the cancers in these patients grow at a slower pace than the cancers in routinely diagnosed patients.

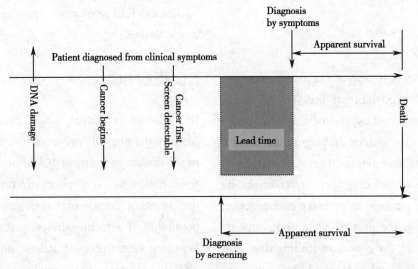

Figure 8-4 A comparison of a patient with a routine clinical diagnosis of disease and a patient with disease detected by screening.

Table 8-8 Criteria for a successful screening program

Basis for Criteria	Criteria
Effect for morbidity and mortality on population	Morbidity or mortality of the disease must be a sufficient concern to public health.
	A high-risk population must exist.
	Effective early intervention must be known to reduce morbidity or mortality.
Screening test	The screening test should be sensitive and specific.
	The screening test must be acceptable to the target population.
	Minimal risk should be associated with the screening.
	Diagnostic workup for a positive test result must have acceptable morbidity given the number of false-positive results.

SUMMARY

In this chapter, the principles of evaluating and interpreting diagnostic tests were introduced. The performance of diagnostic tests can be assessed by accuracy. The first step in the evaluation of a test is determining the "true" status of the disease with gold standard which is considered to represent the true status of disease. **Sensitivity** and **specificity** are terms used to describe the validity of the diagnostic test relative to the gold standard. The sensitivity of a test defined as the percentage of persons with the disease of interest who have positive test results. The greater the sensitivity of a test, the more likely the test will detect persons with the disease of interest. Specificity of a test is defined as the percentage of persons without the disease of interest who have negative test results. The greater the specificity of a test, the more likely it is that persons without the disease of interest will be excluded from consideration of having the disease.

All clinical information is subject to error. One type of error is referred to as a **false-negative** result because the test fails to detect a disease when it is present. A test is said to be **sensitive** when the percentage of false-negative errors is low. A second type of error is referred to as a **false-positive** result because the test indicates that a disease is present when in fact it is not. A test with a low percentage of false-positive results is said to be **specific**.

The performance of diagnostic tests also can be assessed by the use of likelihood ratios. The **likelihood ratio for a positive test** (**LR+**) is the probability of a positive test result for a person with the disease of interest divided by the probability of a positive test result for a person without the disease of interest. The **likelihood ratio for a negative test result** (**LR−**) is the probability of a negative test result for a person with the disease of interest divided by the probability of a negative test result for a person without the disease of interest. LR+ can be used to estimate the posttest probability of disease.

Sensitivity and specificity are characteristics of a diagnostic test. It is useful to consider two other measures, **positive predictive value** (PPV) and **negative predictive value** (NPV), which are used to interpret the results of a diagnostic test. PPV is the percentage of persons with a positive test result who actually have the disease of interest. NPV is the percentage of persons with a negative test result who do not have the disease of interest. Both positive and negative predictive values are heavily influenced by either the pretest probability that the patient has the disease in the particular population that is tested.

For multilevel or continuous outcome test results, a dividing line or **cutoff point** can be chosen to separate findings considered to be positive or negative. Raising the threshold for considering a result to be positive typically will lead to a gain is specificity (fewer false-positive results) but a loss of sensitivity (more false-positive results or missed cases). On the other hand, lowering the threshold for considering a result to be positive typically will reduce the level of false-negative results (raise sensitivity) and increase the likelihood of false-positive results (lower specificity).

The performance of a test can also be represented graphically by a **receiver operating characteristic curve (ROC)**. The area under the ROC curve serves as an overall measure of test performance, with an area of 1 indicating a perfect test and an area of 0.5

indicating a test that is unable to distinguish persons with and without the disease of interest. The respective areas under the ROC curve for two diagnostic tests for a particular disease can be used to identify the test that will provide the greater diagnostic value.

The use of tests to detect the presence of a disease at an earlier time than it would be detected through routine methods is referred to as screening. The evaluation of a screening test must take into account two types of distorting effects: lead-time bias and length-biased sampling.

(Yashuang Zhao)

IMPORTANT TERMINOLOGY

diagnostic test	诊断试验
gold standard	金标准
sensitivity	灵敏度
specificity	特异度
agreement rate	一致率
likelihood ratio	似然比
positive predictive value	阳性预测值
negative predictive value	阴性预测值
receiver operating characteristic curve	受试者工作曲线
serial test	串联试验
parallel test	并联试验
screening	筛检

 STUDY QUESTIONS

1. *In raising the cutoff point for a screening test, which of the following is the likely result?*
   A. *An increase in sensitivity*
   B. *An increase in specificity*
   C. *An increase in false positives*
   D. *An increase in prevalence*
   E. *An increase in lead time bias*

2. *If the screening test does not delay the time of death from a condition but makes survival appear longer because of earlier detection of disease, there is evidence of*
   A. *confounding.*
   B. *length-biased sampling.*
   C. *lead time bias.*
   D. *selection bias.*
   E. *information bias.*

3. *A test with an LR+ of 15 can be said to provide evidence to*
   A. *rule in the condition of interest.*
   B. *rule out the condition of interest.*
   C. *make an earlier diagnosis.*
   D. *prolong survival after diagnosis.*
   E. *detect slowly progressing forms of the condition of interest.*

4. *A specific diagnostic test is one that*
   A. *has a high proportion of false-negative results.*
   B. *has a low proportion of false-negative results.*
   C. *has a high proportion of false-positive results.*
   D. *has a low proportion of false-positive results.*
   E. *none of the above.*

5. *A diagnostic test with no discriminatory ability would have an area under the ROC curve of*
   A. *0.*
   B. *0.25.*
   C. *0.5.*
   D. *1.*
   E. *2.*

6. *A diagnostic test with an LR-of 0.05 can be said to provide evidence to*
   A. *rule in the condition of interest.*
   B. *rule out the condition of interest.*
   C. *make an earlier diagnosis.*
   D. *prolong survival after diagnosis.*
   E. *detect slowly progressing forms of the condition of interest.*

7. *If a screening test does not delay the time of death from a condition but makes survival appear longer because it is preferentially detecting slowly progressing disease, there is evidence of*
   A. *confounding.*
   B. *length-biased sampling.*
   C. *lead time bias.*
   D. *selection bias.*
   E. *information bias.*

8. *Two screening tests are being compared for a particular disease. Test A has an area under the ROC curve of 0.95. Test B has an area under the ROC curve of 0.83. Which of the following statements is correct?*

A. *Neither test has any discriminatory value.*

B. *Test A has a total error rate of 5%.*

C. *Test B is better than test A at ruling in disease.*

D. *The PV+ for test A is 95%.*

E. *Test A performs better than test B at discriminating the presence of disease.*

9. *As the prevalence of a condition increases, a screening test for it will tend to have a*

A. *higher sensitivity.*

B. *higher specificity.*

C. *higher predictive value positive.*

D. *higher predictive value negative.*

E. *higher length biased sampling.*

10. *Which of the following measures of diagnostic test performance ideally has a small value?*

A. *Predictive value positive*

B. *Predictive value negative*

C. *Likelihood ratio for a positive test result*

D. *Likelihood ratio for a negative test result*

E. *None of the above*

FURTHER READING

Lichtman JH, Bigger JT Jr, Blumenthal JA, et al.American Heart Association Prevention Committee of the Council on Cardiovascular Nursing; American Heart Association Council on Clinical Cardiology; American Heart Association Council on Epidemiology and Prevention; American Heart Association Interdisciplinary Council on Quality of Care and Outcomes Research; American Psychiatric Association. Depression and coronary heart disease: recommendations for screening, referral, and treatment. A science advisory from the American Heart Association Prevention Committee of the Council on Cardiovascular Nursing, Council on Clinical Cardiology, Council on Epidemiology and Prevention, and Interdisciplinary Council on Quality of Care and Outcomes Research. *Circulation.* 2008;118:1768-1775.

Lichtman JH, Froelicher ES, Blumenthal JA, et al.American Heart Association Statistics Committee of the Council on Epidemiology and Prevention and the Council on Cardio-

vascular and Stroke Nursing. Depression as a risk factor for poor prognosis among patients with acute coronary syndrome: systematic review and recommendations: a scientific statement from the American Heart Association. *Circulation.* 2014;129:1350-1369.

Thombs BD, Roseman M, Coyne JC, et al. Does evidence support the American Heart Association's recommendation to screen patients for depression in cardiovascular care? An updated systematic review. *PLoS ONE.* 2013;8:e52654.

REFERENCE

Raymon S Greenberg. Medical Epidemiology. 5th ed. Population Health and Effective Health Care, Chapter 10 of-Diagnostic Testing. *Mc Graw Hill Education.* April 2015; 127-139.

Sensitivity and Specificity

Elderon L, Smolderen KG, Na B, et al. Accuracy and prognostic value of American Heart Association— recommended depression screening in patients with coronary heart disease: data from the Heart and Soul Study. *Circ Cardiovasc Qual Outcomes.* 2011;4:533-540.

Positive and Negative Predictive Value
Cutoff Points

Zuithoff NPA, Vergouwe Y, King M, et al. The Patient Health Questionnaire-9 for detection of major depressive disorder in primary care: consequences of current thresholds in a cross-sectional study. *BMC Family Pract.* 2010;11:98.

Likelihood Ratios

Elderon L, Smolderen KG, Na B, Whooley MA. Accuracy and prognostic value of American Heart Association— recommended depression screening in patients with coronary heart disease: data from the Heart and Soul Study. Circ Cardiovasc Qual Outcomes.2011;4:533-540.

ROC Curves

Zuithoff NPA, Vergouwe Y, King M, et al. The Patient Health Questionnaire-9 for detection of major depressive disorder in primary care: consequences of current thresholds in a cross-sectional study. BMC Family Pract. 2010;11:98.

9 Variability and Bias

HEALTH SCENARIO

A 45-year-old man began working as a production supervisor, and his employer required that he undergo a complete medical examination. His physician learned that the patient's father had died of myocardial infarction at age 65. On physical examination, the patient was moderately obese, and his blood pressure was 140/86 mmHg. The remainder of the examination revealed no notable abnormalities. The patient's total serum cholesterol level (nonfasting) was 242 mg/dl.

According to the Chinese Medical Association (CMA) Guideline for Blood Lipids Abnormality Prevention for Chinese Adults, a total serum cholesterol concentration over 240 mg/dl is an indication for possible pharmacologic lowering of serum cholesterol. A value of 220-239 mg/dl is considered borderline and should trigger life-style change, e.g., dietary intervention, and a value less than 220 mg/dl is considered normal.

Based on the initial cholesterol results, the physician asked the patient to return in 2 weeks for further testing. On repeat measurement, the total serum cholesterol concentration was 198 mg/dl on a fasting lipid profile. Table 9-1 lists several different factors that could explain the observed variability in measured total serum cholesterol level. The source of this variability in the measured total cholesterol level had important implications for how the physician treated his patient.

VARIABILITY IN MEDICAL RESEARCH

Difficulties in the interpretation of test results of individual patient are magnified when groups of patients are studied. The sources of **variability** in test results and errors in medical research are discussed in this chapter. Appreciation of these issues is important for the interpretation and appropriate application of research findings in the clinical setting.

Table 9-1 Levels of variability.

Levels	Features
Individual	Individual variability
	Measurement variability
Population	Genetic variability between individuals
	Environmental variability
	Measurement variability
Sample	Manner of sampling
	Size of sample
	Measurement variability

Variability in measurements can be either random or systematic. A schematic representation of random and systematic variation is shown in Figure 9-1. The shots at the targets in both A and B are centered around the middle, but in A the shots are less scattered and have less variability, or more precision. In targets C and D the scatter is similar, but in target D the cluster of shots is off center. This might occur, for example, if the sight of the gun were bent. The precision is comparable, but the result in D is systematically off target or biased. The results in target C are accurate, or valid. It is important to consider the accuracy and precision of any measurements made in the medical setting. In clinical medicine and medical research, variability can occur at a number of different levels (eg, at the level of the individual or the population) (Table 9-1). At each level, the variability inherent in the method of measurement is important.

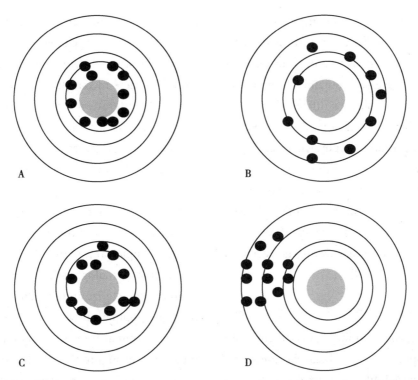

Figure 9-1. Schematic illustrations of increased random error (target *B* versus target *A*) and systematic error (target *D* versus target *C*).

Variability Within the Individual

The first level of concern is variability in the true value of a person's characteristics over time. This was a source of concern for the clinician in the Case Example. Some potential sources of individual variability are listed in Table 9-2. Variation can occur because of biological changes in an individual over time. These changes may (1) occur on a minute-to-minute basis (eg, heart rate), (2) follow a regular diurnal pattern (eg, body temperature), or (3) progress with normal development (eg, height or weight).

When the variation within a subject is large, a single measurement may not adequately represent the "true" status of that individual. By repeating a test, the physician may obtain a better understanding of the true value and its variability. This may also provide the clinician with information about variability or error due to the measurement technique. In the Case Example, different results were obtained when the total serum cholesterol level was measured a second time—when the patient was fasting. It is unlikely, however, that the fasting state alone could cause such a drop in total serum cholesterol concen-

tration. Furthermore, it is unlikely that the patient could have made the kind of dietary or other alterations in 2 weeks that would lead to the observed changes in total serum cholesterol level.

Table 9-2 Potential sources of variability in measurements of individuals.

Sources of variability	Features
Individual characteristics	Diurnal variation
	Changes related to factors such as age, diet, and exercise
	Environmental factors such as season or temperature
Measurement characteristics	Poor calibration of instrument
	Inherent lack of precision of the instrument
	Misreading or misrecording information from the instrument by the technician

Variability Related to Measurement

Laboratory measurements of total serum cholesterol level are notorious for both variability and error. To determine which value 198 mg/dl or 242 mg/dl is closer to the truth, the physician in the Case Example would need to know whether both measurements were obtained in the same laboratory. For example, the first result may have been obtained from a desktop analyzer in the physician's office, whereas the lipid profile may have been measured in a standardized laboratory. In reality, the physician may not be able to discern readily which value is closer to the truth. This is one reason that programs with guidelines that support cutoff points for clinical decision making often recommend that elevated values be confirmed by repeated measurements over time before treatment is instituted.

Variations Within Populations

Just as there is variability in individuals, there is also variability in populations, which can be considered the cumulative variability of individuals. Because populations are made up of individuals with different genetic constitutions who are subject to different environmental influences, populations often exhibit more variation than individuals. Physicians use knowledge about variability in populations to define what is "normal" and "abnormal". The physician in the Case Example could refer to population survey data to learn that for 45-year-old males, a total serum cholesterol level of 200 mg/dl is close to the 50th percentile, and a concentration of 240 mg/dl is equivalent to the 75th percentile. Accordingly, the patient generally falls in the upper half of the population distribution of total serum cholesterol values. Assuming that the measurement is correct, this could be a result of genetic factors, environmental factors, or both.

Variability in Research Studies

It is worthwhile to ask how the clinician would know that a total serum cholesterol value in the upper end of the population distribution is disadvantageous. Do these values really indicate unhealthy? Answers may be found in studies that have linked the level of total serum cholesterol with an increased risk of cardiovascular mortality. In cohort studies such as the Framingham Heart Study, groups of subjects were

followed and compared according to their different levels of total serum cholesterol and the associated frequency of death from myocardial infarction or stroke. In these investigations, a higher level of total serum cholesterol was associated with an increased risk of death from cardiovascular disease.

When investigators perform such studies, they cannot usually study the entire population. Instead they study subsets or samples of the population. This introduces another source of variability-sampling variability-that is important in medical research. Using a single sample of subjects to represent the population is analogous to using a single measurement to characterize an individual. Repeated samples from the population will give different estimates of the true population values. Sampling variability is illustrated in Figure 9-2. In the source population of 20 persons, there are five individuals (25%) with total serum cholesterol values above 240 mg/dl. In the three different samples of five subjects drawn from the source population by chance, the proportion of individuals with total serum cholesterol val-

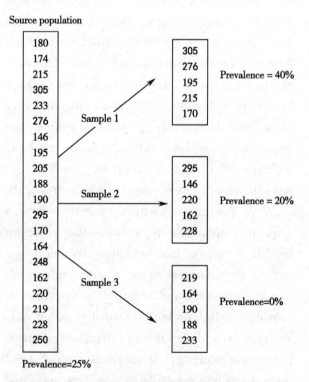

Figure 9-2. Schematic diagram of sampling variability. The source population of 20 persons has a 25% prevalence of hypercholesterolemia (elevated cholesterol values are presented in bold). The three random samples of five persons yield prevalence estimates ranging from 0 to 40%.

ues above 240 mg/dl ranges from 0 to 40%. Each of these small samples presents a different picture of the source population. A larger sample size would result in less variability and would more likely represent the source population.

Variability can be important in other ways when two groups are compared in a study. The goal of such studies often is to determine whether a measurable difference exists between the groups. When a research paper reports no statistically significant differences between groups, the reader must ask the following questions: Was there actually no difference between the two treatments, or was the estimate of effect so imprecise that the investigator could not distinguish difference between the two groups (i.e., a type II error)?

A graphic display of the results of two hypothetic studies of the same question is presented in Figure 9-3. In each study, the investigators attempted to determine whether a cholesterol-lowering drug had a favorable effect on the risk of developing myocardial infarction. The measure of effect that was estimated in each study was the risk ratio. Each study compared a group of patients randomly allocated to receive the cholesterol-lowering drug with a group chosen to receive dietary modification alone. The researchers reached different conclusions. In the study with the smaller sample, the report indicated that the drug had no beneficial effect on reducing the risk of developing myocardial infarction, when compared with diet therapy. In the study with the larger sample, the

investigators concluded that the drug decreased the risk of developing myocardial infarction, when compared with dietary management.

As shown in Figure 9-3, Study A has a small sample size, which resulted in imprecise estimates (i.e., wide confidence intervals) of the risk of developing myocardial infarction in the two groups. Consequently, the two estimates overlapped, and the statistical test was not capable of distinguishing between the effects of the two treatments. The investigators concluded that there was no difference in risk of developing myocardial infarction between patients who received cholesterol-lowering drug and dietary therapy. In Study B, the investigator used a larger sample size yielding the same point estimates of risk in the two groups but with much greater precision (i.e., narrower confidence intervals) in the estimate of the effects of the drug. With this gain in precision, the statistical test was able to distinguish between the two groups, and the investigator was able to infer correctly that the cholesterol-lowering drug was superior to dietary therapy. Generally, the larger the sample size, the more precise the estimate of effect and the smaller the detectable differences between groups. In studies with very large sample sizes, small differences between groups may be judged to be statistically significant but have little biological or clinical meaning. For example, a study of 20,000 subjects might have concluded that a 1% difference in risk of developing myocardial infarction was statistically significant. It is unlikely, however, that a difference

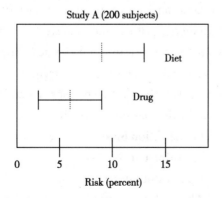
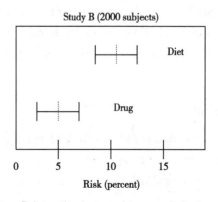

Figure 9-3. The effect of sample size on precision of risk estimates. Point estimates are shown as dashed vertical lines and 95% confidence interval are shown as solid horizontal lines. In both studies, the 5-year risk of developing myocardial infarction was 9% among persons receiving dietary therapy and 6% among persons treated with a cholesterol-lowering drug. In the larger study, however, the 95% confidence intervals are narrower, and the difference in risk between treatment groups is statistically significant.

in risk this small would justify prolonged use of the cholesterol-lowering agent.

VALIDITY

*The concept of **validity** concerns the degree to which a measurement or study reaches a correct conclusion.* A measurement or study may lead to an incorrect (invalid) conclusion because of the effects of bias. The variability seen with bias is systematic or nonrandom and distorts the estimated effect. In Figure 9-1, the amount of bias can be determined by the degree to which the shots are off target in *D*. Unfortunately, in medical research the truth (bull's-eye) may not be known, or there may be no "gold standard" for comparison. Consequently, the degree of bias often is difficult to determine. Two different types of validity, internal validity and external validity, are described in this chapter.

Internal Validity

***Internal validity** is the extent to which the results of an investigation accurately reflect the true situation of the study population.* If the results are not valid in the study population, there is little reason to suspect that those results will apply to other populations. Internal validity is defined by the boundaries of the study itself. Therefore, a study is internally valid if it provides a true estimate of effect, given the limits of the population studied. Measures that can be used to improve internal validity often involve restricting the type of subjects and the environment in which the study is performed. These measures decrease the impact of factors extraneous to the question of interest.

External Validity

A result obtained in a tightly controlled environment, however, may not be applicable to more general situations. ***External validity** is the extent to which the results of a study are applicable to other populations.* External validity addresses the following question: Do these results apply to other patients, such as patients who are older, sicker, or less economically advantaged than subjects in the study?

External validity often is of particular interest to clinicians who must decide if a research finding is applicable to their clinical practice. Determining whether the results of a study can be generalized involves a judgment regarding the following:

(1) The type of subjects included in the investigation;

(2) The type of patients seen by the clinician;

(3) Whether there are clinically meaningful differences between the study population and other populations.

An example of the kind of difficulty that can occur when study results are generalized is the criticism that too many clinical studies focus on males. One such study is the Lipid Research Clinics-Primary Prevention Trial, which demonstrated a significant reduction on cardiovascular mortality for white men aged 35-59 years with hypercholesterolemia who were placed on a cholesterol-lowering diet and medication. Do the results also apply to women? Do they apply to men of different ages, races, or with different, but still abnormal, serum cholesterol levels? These questions led to the suggestion that efforts should be made to include women, minorities, and children in the study populations.

Bias

***Bias** is a systematic error in a study that leads to a distortion of the results.* Bias, a threat to validity, can occur in any research, but is of particular concern in observational studies because the lack of randomization increases the chance that study groups will differ with respect to important characteristics. Bias often is subdivided into different categories, based on how bias enters the study. The most common classification divides bias into three categories:

(1) **Selection bias;**

(2) **Information bias;**

(3) **Confounding.**

Although these categories overlap, this classification is useful because it provides the reader with a systematic approach to evaluate bias. It should be remembered that with the exception of confounding, which can be quantitated, the evaluation of bias is subjective and involves a judgment regarding the likelihood of (1) the presence of bias and (2) its direction and potential magnitude of effect on the results. Even though the magnitude of bias cannot be quantified, often its influence on the results of a study can be inferred. It is important to discern whether the suspected bias is likely to make an association appear stronger or weaker than it really is. Overestimation of a risk ratio for a protective exposure and a separate hazardous exposure is demonstrated schematically in Figure 9-4. Underestimation of a risk ratio for a protective exposure and a hazard-

ous exposure is shown in Figure 9-5.

Selection Bias

A variety of procedures can be used to select subjects for a study. Usually, it is not possible to include all individuals with a particular disease or exposure in a study, so a sample of subjects must be chosen. The procedures used for the selection of subjects depend on a number of factors, including

(1) The design of the investigation;

(2) The setting of the study;

(3) The disease and exposure of interest.

Often subjects are selected in a manner that is

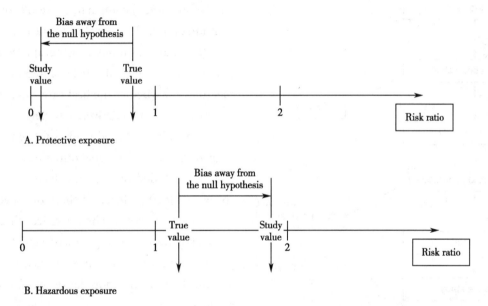

Figure 9-4. Overestimation of a risk ratio for (A) a protective exposure and (B) a hazardous exposure.

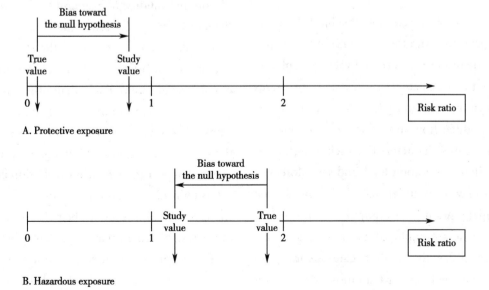

Figure 9-5. Underestimation of a risk ratio for (A) a protective exposure and (B) a hazardous exposure.

convenient for the investigator. Under optimal circumstances, the method for inclusion of subjects leads to a valid comparison that, in turn, yields correct information regarding a disease process or treatment. The selection process itself, however, may increase or decrease the chance that a relationship between the exposure and disease of interest will be detected. A schematic diagram of the steps involved in recruiting and maintaining a study population is shown in Figure 9-6. From this diagram, it is easy to see that selection factors could lead to biased results at several different steps in the process.

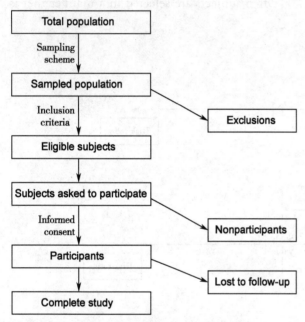

Figure 9-6. Steps in the selection and maintenance of subjects in a study.

Some aspects of the selection of subjects lead primarily to problems with the generalization (extrapolation) of the results (i.e., external validity). Subjects must agree to participate in a study, and this causes one of the most common problems. Volunteers for a study may differ from individuals who do not volunteer in various characteristics such as age, race, economic status, education level, and sex. Moreover, volunteers may be healthier than those who decline to participate. A study of a population limited to individuals who are employed may also make it difficult to generalize the result, because people who work are generally healthier than those who do not. A comparison of health outcomes between workers

and the general population may show that the workers have a more favorable outcome simply because they are healthy enough to be employed (the "healthy worker" effect).

Referral of patients to clinical facilities can also lead to distorted study conclusions. Selective referral patterns can be seen in the study of children with febrile seizures. Febrile seizures are brief, generalized seizures that occur in conjunction with elevation in temperature in children aged 6 months to 6 years. There is some disagreement about whether these febrile convulsions are predictive of future seizures and other unfavorable neurologic sequelae. Ellenberg and Nelson (1980) compared the results of a number of studies on the long-term outcome of patients with febrile seizures. Studies of geographically defined populations in which affected children were followed, regardless of whether medical care was sought, consistently revealed a relatively low rate of unfavorable sequelae. Clinical-based studies tended to report a high frequency of adverse outcomes. Accordingly, it was concluded that clinical-based studies selectively included children at the more severe end of the clinical spectrum. The inferences that might be drawn regarding the prognosis of a child with febrile seizures might be very different based on whether a clinical-based or a population-based sample was studied.

Other aspects of the selection process can diminish internal validity. *In a clinical trial or cohort study, the major potential selection bias is loss to follow-up.* Once subjects are enrolled in the study, they may decide to discontinue participation. Certain types of subjects are more likely than others to drop out of a study. Furthermore, during the course of the study some subjects may die from causes other than the outcome of interest. At first glance, these losses may not appear to be related to selection because the subject already was enrolled in the study. If the lost subjects differ, however, in their risk of the outcome of interest, biased estimates of risk may be obtained.

If the unrecognized early manifestations of the disease of interest cause exposed persons to leave the study more or less frequently than unexposed persons, a distorted conclusion might be reached. For example, in a randomized controlled trial of the effects of using a cholesterol-lowering drug versus diet therapy on prevention of myocardial infarctions, bias might be introduced if drug-treated patients with coronary insufficiency were more likely to develop side effects from treatment and withdrew from participation, whereas patients with coronary insufficiency receiving dietary therapy remained in the study.

Selection bias is of particular importance in case-control studies (see Chapter 6) in which the investigator must select two study groups, cases and controls, in a setting in which the exposure has already occurred. For example, it must be decided whether to use existing (prevalent) cases who are available at the time of study, regardless of the duration of their disease, or to limit eligibility to newly diagnosed (incident) cases. If the risk factor of interest also is a prognostic factor, the use of prevalent cases can lead to a biased conclusion. Consider, for example, a case-control study of total serum cholesterol level as a risk factor for developing myocardial infarction. Suppose that of patients who have a myocardial infarction those with very high total serum cholesterol levels are more likely to die suddenly than those with lower serum cholesterol levels. Under these circumstances, a comparison of patients surviving myocardial infarction with controls will underestimate the true association between elevation in total serum cholesterol level and risk of developing myocardial infarction.

Another potential type of selection bias can occur when a case-control study involves subjects who are hospitalized. Patients with two medical conditions are more likely to be hospitalized than those with a single disease. Thus, a hospital-based case-control study might find a link between two diseases or between an exposure and a disease when there is no association between them in the general population. This type of bias, often called Berkson's bias, was demonstrated in a study that showed that respiratory and bone diseases were associated in a sample of hospitalized patients but not in the general population.

Thus, in a hospital-based study, an exposure such as cigarette smoking, which is correlated with respiratory disease, may also appear to occur together with bone disease because those diseases are related in hospitalized patients.

Information bias

Information (or misclassification) bias can occur when there is random or systematic inaccuracy in measurement. This can be visualized best in epidemiological studies that involve dichotomous exposure and disease variables, such as elevated total serum cholesterol and myocardial infarction. Subjects are classified according to whether they have had high total serum cholesterol levels and whether they have had a myocardial infarction. The investigator either can be correct or incorrect, resulting in true-positive and true-negative findings, as well as false-positive and false-negative classifications of subjects with respect to either exposure or disease.

If the errors in classification of exposure or disease status are independent of the level of the other variable, then the misclassification is termed nondifferential. **Nondifferential misclassification** may occur in a case-control study if the subject's memory of exposure status is unrelated to whether the subject has the disease of interest. An example of nondifferential misclassification is sometimes referred to as unacceptability bias. Subjects may answer a question about the exposure with a socially acceptable but sometimes inaccurate response, regardless of whether they have the disease of interest. Consider a case-control study of myocardial infarction in which the exposure of interest is prior intake of foods high in saturated fats. Regardless of disease status, respondents may underreport intake of foods with high fat content because they think low-fat diets are more acceptable to the investigator. In most instances, when nondifferential misclassification occurs, it blurs differences between the study groups, making it more difficult for the investigator to detect a real association between the exposure and the disease. This is often referred to as a bias toward the null hypothesis or toward no association.

Differential misclassification occurs when the misclassification of one variable depends on the status of the other. In a case-control study, this type of misclassification could occur if the information on exposure status depends on whether the subject has the disease. If a case with a myocardial infarction is more likely to overestimate the level of dietary fat intake than a control subject, a biased result may occur. In this instance, the bias would lead to an overestimate of the relationship between dietary fat intake and risk of developing myocardial infarction.

The difference between nondifferential and differential misclassification can be demonstrated by examining the data in Figure 9-7. Consider a case-control study of the relationship between high-fat diets and risk of developing myocardial infarction in which the true odds ratio (*OR*) is 2.3. With nondifferential misclassification, the subjects did not recall the amount of fatty foods eaten, but the errors in recall did not depend on whether they had a myocardial infarction. In this situation, 20% of both cases and controls who ate high-fat diets underreported fat intake. The resulting *OR* of 2.0 was an underestimate of the true *OR*. On the other hand, if all the patients who had a myocardial infarction correctly recalled

their dietary fat exposure status, but only 80% of the exposed controls correctly reported their exposure, then **differential misclassification** would occur. This type of misclassification can result in either an underestimate or overestimate of the true OR. In this example, the investigator overestimated the OR.

Two common types of differential information bias are often referred to as **recall bias** and **interviewer bias**. Recall bias results from differential ability of subjects to remember previous activities and exposures. Patients who have a serious disease may search their memory for an exposure in an attempt to explain or to understand why they acquired the illness. Control subjects, who do not have the disease, may be less likely to remember an exposure because it has less meaning and is less important for them.

When interviewers are employed to determine exposures in case-control studies, results may be influenced by how the interviewers collect information. If they are aware of the research hypothesis, the interviewers intentionally or unintentionally may influence the responses of the subjects. They may probe more deeply for responses from cases than from controls. If a dietary exposure is examined, the interviewers may ask certain subjects specific ques-

Nondifferential misclassification

Truth:	Dietary fat	
	High	Low
MI	60	40
No MI	40	60

OR=(60 × 60)/(40 × 40)=2.3

Study:	Dietary fat	
	High	Low
MI	48	52
No MI	32	68

OR=(48 × 68)/(52 × 32)=2.0

Differential misclassification

Truth:	Dietary fat	
	High	Low
MI	60	40
No MI	40	60

OR=(60 × 60)/(40 × 40)=2.3

Study:	Dietary fat	
	High	Low
MI	60	40
No MI	32	68

OR=(60 × 68)/(40 × 32)=3.2

Figure 9-7. Illustration of nondifferential and differential misclassification of exposure to high-fat diets in a case-control study of myocardial infarction(MI). (OR=odds ratio)

tions about particular food items. Interviewers may also give the subjects subtle clues by tone of voice or body language that suggest a preference for certain responses. Generally, it is desirable to blind the interviewers to the research hypothesis under investigation.

In a case-control study, however, it may be difficult to blind the interviewers to the disease status of cases and controls. Nevertheless, if the interviewers are not aware of the exposure of primary interest, biased data collection still can be minimized.

As a way to reduce misclassification and to improve accuracy of study measurements, investigators increasingly are using **biological markers**. As shown in Table 9-3, these markers can measure many facets of disease and exposure—or the relationship between the two. For example, biological markers can measure:

(1) Susceptibility (biological markers can be used to identify subjects with particularly high risk due to a particular biological predisposition);

(2) Internal dose (biological markers can be used to measure the amount of a chemical or other exposure in the body);

(3) Biologically effective dose (biological markers can be used to measure the amount of a substance that reaches the target sites);

(4) Biological effect (biological markers can be used to quantify a deleterious effect of a particular exposure).

Biological markers are used in most substantive areas of investigation, including nutritional, cardiovascular, reproductive, cancer, and infectious disease epidemiology. Use of biological markers is important in observational studies for several reasons. These markers are important methodologically because they can serve to reduce misclassification by allowing more accurate assessment of exposure or disease status. Furthermore, they may allow the investigator to define more homogeneous disease categories or to identify susceptible subjects, so that the study can focus on specific subgroups.

Finally, biological markers can help provide insight into the underlying disease process and pathogenesis.

Table 9-3 Uses of biological markers in epidemiology

Application of Marker	Example
To measure susceptibility	Those with high aryl hydrocarbon hydoxylase activity have higher risk of bladder cancer
To measure internal dose	Those with high serum carotene levels may have lower risk of lung cancer
To measure biologically effective dose	Those with greater amounts of effective dose of polycyclic aromatic hydrocarbon-DNA adducts have experienced greater exposure and interaction of their DNA to these carcinogenic hydrocarbons[a]
To measure biological effect	Higher levels of the *ras* oncogene product may be a preclinical marker of early carcinogenic response[a]

[a] Perera F et al: Biologic markers in risk assessment for environmental carcinogens. Environ Health Persp 1991; 90:247.

The use of levels of serum dioxin to measure exposure of men who worked with the herbicide Agent Orange during the Vietnam War illustrates the use of a biological marker to measure internal dose. After the Vietnam War, concern arose about wartime exposures of servicemen to Agent Orange, in part because of its contamination with the highly toxic trace contaminant known as 2,3,7,8-tetrachlorodibenzo-p-dioxin (TCDD). Because of this concern, Air Force researchers began epidemiologic studies to assess the health effects among Air Force veterans associated with exposure to Agent Orange and TCDD. Researchers initially used job descriptions to classify exposure to TCDD. Later, after laboratory techniques became available to measure minute concentrations of TCDD within the blood, the researchers discovered that classification of exposure based on job descriptions was associated with substantial misclassification. In subsequent studies, the more accurate serum TCDD measurements were used to assess exposures.

Despite the importance of biological markers and the possibility that their use may reduce information bias, they do not eliminate the possibility of systematic errors. Although it may be diminished by employing a biological marker, misclassification remains a possibility. For example, marker instability and inter- or intra-individual variability can contribute to measurement errors. Moreover, if required biological specimens are collected after disease occurrence, as often happens in case-control studies, the presence of disease in cases may affect the biological marker. This possibility can make the biological marker particularly susceptible to differential misclassification and measurement error. Bias can even be created if the investigator adjusts inappropriately for a factor that is caused by the exposure of interest and is associated with the outcome.

Case-control studies of the relationship of β-carotene and cancer illustrate the potential for residual information bias. β-Carotene is a fat-soluble antioxidant found in many fruits and vegetables. It acts as a provitamin (vitamin A), protects against development of cancer in animals, and may reduce the risk of developing cancer in humans. In a case-control study of serum levels of this antioxidant, differential misclassification could create or accentuate a protective effect, if cases with advanced cancer had altered nutritional status and a resulting lowering of β-carotene levels. Although these biases are somewhat speculative, the potential for bias in case-control studies is evident.

Thus, use of biological markers offers many advantages, particularly an improved assessment of exposure and a more homogeneous definition of disease. Nevertheless, because use of these markers does not eliminate the possibility of information bias, caution in interpretation is still warranted.

Confounding

Confounding refers to the mixing of the effect of an extraneous variable with the effects of the exposure and disease of interest. Confounding can be demonstrated by the following hypothetical example. Suppose investigators undertake a case-control study of the association between high total serum cholesterol level and risk of developing myocardial infarction. From the results of other studies, the researchers know that the risk of myocardial infarction is asso-

ciated with obesity, and that total cholesterol levels also correlate with obesity (see Figure 9-8). Suppose that in our hypothetical case-control study, 36 of 60 patients with myocardial infarction (60%) are found to have high total serum cholesterol levels, and only 24 of 60 controls (40%) are discovered to have elevated serum cholesterol levels. This would suggest that elevated total serum cholesterol levels are associated with an increased risk of developing myocardial infarction.

When the observed association is examined separately in obese and nonobese persons, however, a different conclusion is reached. Among obese persons, 34 of 40 patients with myocardial infarction (85%) and 18 of 20 controls (90%) are found to have elevated total serum cholesterol levels. Among nonobese persons, 2 of 20 patients with myocardial infarction (10%) and 6 of 40 controls (15%) have high total serum cholesterol levels. Thus, in the case of both obese and nonobese individuals, elevated total serum cholesterol levels are more common in controls than in patients with myocardial infarction. Keep in mind that in the hypothetical study, obesity was associated with myocardial infarction, since 52 of 60 obese subjects (87%) had elevated total serum cholesterol levels, and only 8 of 60 nonobese persons (13%) had high total serum cholesterol levels. Clearly, in this hypothetical example, the results are confounded by the extraneous variable, obesity. The results are illustrated in Figure 9-9.

For a variable—in this case, obesity—to be considered a potential confounder, it must satisfy two conditions:

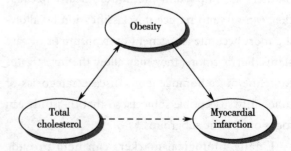

Figure 9-8. Schematic diagram of the relationship between total serum cholesterol level and risk of developing myocardial infarction, with confounding by obesity.

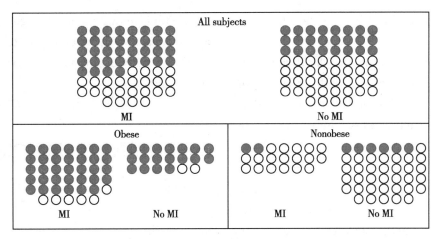

Figure 9-9. Illustration of the relationship between total serum cholesterol level and risk of developing myocardial infarction (MI), with confounding by obesity. Shaded circles represent persons with elevated total serum cholesterol levels and unshaded circles represent persons with normal total serum cholesterol levels.

(1) Association with the disease of interest in the absence of exposure;

(2) Association with the exposure but not as a result of being exposed.

Because it can be evaluated in the analysis of results, confounding differs from selection bias and information bias. The presence of confounding is demonstrated by a change in the apparent strength of association between the exposure and the disease of interest when the effects of extraneous variables are taken into account. Confounding, which is not an all-or-none property of an extraneous variable, may occur to different degrees in different studies.

Generally, the list of potential confounders in a study is limited to established risk factors for the disease of interest. There are two accepted methods for dealing with potential confounders. The first is to consider them in the design of the study by matching on the potential confounder or by restricting the sample to limited levels of the potential confounder. The other method is to evaluate confounding in the analysis by stratification, as demonstrated schematically in Figure 9-9, or by using multivariate analysis techniques such as multiple logistic regression.

The goal of any epidemiologic study is to provide a valid conclusion. To accomplish this objective, complete attention must be given to all aspects of the study, from inception to design and data collection and, finally, to analysis and reporting of results. It is important to remember that bias can be introduced

at any of these stages, leading to erroneous results. Thus, it is useful to look carefully for potential sources of bias and to consider their possible impact. Clinicians must judge whether results can be generalized to their particular practice. Understanding the potential problems with measurement and bias in medical research improves the ability of physicians to decide on appropriate preventive and therapeutic strategies.

SUMMARY

In this chapter, the topics of variability and systematic errors in epidemiologic measurements are discussed, with illustrative examples that focus primarily on the relationship between total serum cholesterol level and the risk of developing myocardial infarction. A distinction is drawn between random variation, which is inversely related to precision in measurement, and nonrandom or systematic error, which is related to a distortion in measurement.

Variability can arise from (1) the subjects under study, (2) differences between individuals, (3) the approach used to sample subjects, or (4) the measurement process itself. Variability related to sampling is likely to diminish as the sample size increases. With extremely large sample sizes, a very small difference in outcome between study groups can be statistically significant. Whether the magnitude of this difference is sufficient to warrant a change in clinical practice is a separate, but equally important, question.

Validity concerns the extent to which the findings of a study reflect truth. **Internal validity** relates to the accuracy of study findings for the persons who are investigated. **External validity** concerns the extent to which study findings accurately apply to persons who are not studied.

Bias is defined as lack of validity. Conventionally, bias is classified into three major types: **selection bias, information (misclassification) bias,** and **confounding.** Selection bias refers to the introduction of systematic errors into study results through the manner in which study subjects are selected. Information bias results in systematic errors in study findings that originate in the approach to collecting information. Two kinds of information bias can exist. **Nondifferential misclassification** occurs when errors in the information about one variable are unrelated to the status of another variable. **Differential misclassification,** on the other hand, occurs when errors in the information about one variable are affected by the status of another variable.

Confounding is concerned with the mixing of the primary effect of interest with the effects of one or more extraneous factors. In experimental studies, the problem of confounding is reduced by randomization, which tends to balance the study groups with respect to both known and unknown determinants of the outcome. In observational research, however, study groups may differ appreciably in factors that are (1) related to the risk of disease among unexposed persons and (2) are also associated with the exposure of interest, but not as a result of being exposed. The influence of these potential confounders can be addressed in the study design (eg, through matching or restrictive inclusion criteria) or in the analysis (eg, through stratification or regression techniques). Only known confounders can be addressed in observational research.

No study is immune from the possibility of bias. The investigator must therefore consider potential sources of bias when sampling subjects, collecting information, analyzing results, and interpreting findings. With planning and forethought, it is possible to anticipate and avoid certain types of error and thus conduct a study that leads to a convincing and valid conclusion.

(Zhijiang Zhang)

IMPORTANT TERMINOLOGY

variability	变异性
validity	真实性
internal validity	内部真实性
external validity	外部真实性
bias	偏倚
selection bias	选择偏倚
information bias	信息偏倚
nondifferential misclassification	无差异性错误分类
differential misclassification	差异性错误分类
confounding	混杂

 STUDY QUESTIONS

Questions 1-3: For each numbered situation below, select from the following lettered options the type of error that would most likely result. Each option can be used once, more than once, or not at all.

A. *Selection bias*

B. *Nondifferential misclassification*

C. *Differential misclassification*

D. *Confounding*

E. *Random error*

1. *In a case-control study of the relationship between a cholesterol lowering drug and the risk of developing breast cancer, control subjects are sampled from participants in a health screening fair.*

2. *In a cohort study of hormone replacement therapy and the risk of developing atherosclerotic coronary artery disease, high socioeconomic status is associated with both use of hormone replacement therapy and the risk of developing coronary artery disease.*

3. *In a case-control study of the relationship of stressful life events and the occurrence of coronary artery disease, the cases are more likely than the controls to overreport stressful events.*

Questions 4-5: For each numbered situation below,

select from the following lettered options the most likely effect on the study findings. Each option can be used once, more than once, or not at all.

A. Overestimation

B. Underestimation

C. No effect

D. Cannot be determined

4. In a cohort study of obesity and the risk of developing non-insulin-dependent diabetes mellitus, the loss to follow-up is greater for obese compared to nonobese persons.

5. In a case-control study of ingestion of L-tryptophan as a risk factor for developing eosinophilia-myalgia syndrome (EMS), women with EMS tend to give more false-positive reports of using L-tryptophan than do women without EMS.

REFERENCES

Case Example

The joint committee for revision of the dislipidemia management guidetine for Chinese adult. A guideline for the dyslipidemia management in Chinese adult (2016 revision). Chincse Circulation Journal. 2016;10:937.

Variability Related to Measurement

Report of the National Cholesterol Education Program Expert Panel on detection, evaluation and treatment of high blood cholesterol in adults. *Arch Intern Med*. 1988;148:36.

External Validity

Altman DG, Bland JM.Generalization and extrapolation.*BMJ* 1998;317:409.

Lipid Research Clinic Program.The Lipid Research Clinic's Coronary Primary Prevention Trial results. 1. Reduction in incidence of coronary heart disease. *JAMA*. 1984;251:351.

Selection Bias

Ellenberg JH, Nelson KB.Sample selection and the natural history of disease: Studies of febrile seizures. *JAMA*. 1980;243:1337.

Roberts RS, Spitzer WO, Delmore T, et al. Empirical demonstration of Berkson's bias. *J Chron Dis*. 1978; 31:119.

Information Bias

Coates RJ, et al.Cancer risk in relation to serum copper levels. *Cancer Res*. 1989;49:4353.

Hulka BS, Wilcosky TC, Griffith JD: *Biologic Markers in Epidemiology*. Oxford University Press, 1990.

Perera F, et al. Biologic markers in risk assessment for environmental carcinogens. *Environ Health Persp*.1991; 90:247.

Confounding

Weinberg CR.Toward a clearer definition of confounding. *Am J Epidemiol*. 1993; 137:1.

PATIENT PROFILE

A 40-year-old accountant visited her family physician for a routine checkup. The patient's mother had been diagnosed with breast cancer in the past year, and the patient wanted advice about what she could do to reduce her own risk of developing this disease. The patient had two children, aged 6 and 8 years. She was in good health, with regular menstrual cycles, and she had a recent normal Papanicolaou smear and mammogram.

In responding to the patient's questions about breast cancer, the physician confirmed that a positive family history increases the risk of developing this disease. A number of other characteristics are associated with a reduced risk of developing breast cancer, such as early age at first full-term pregnancy and an increasing number of pregnancies. Unfortunately, these factors are not easily susceptible to intervention, and the patient had already completed her childbearing. The physician was also aware of a controversy regarding dietary fat intake and the occurrence of breast cancer. Before recommending that the patient reduce her fat intake, however, the physician wished to review the pertinent medical literature.

INTRODUCTION

The recommendations that physicians make to patients depend on the current state of available knowledge about diseases, the underlying pathophysiology of diseases, and the most effective treatment for diseases. The knowledge base of clinical medicine is continuously expanding, and physicians must therefore develop methods to seek out and apply new information. This process is complicated when inconclusive or conflicting results are found in the medical literature. The publication of articles, even in the most respected journals, does not guarantee that the investigators' conclusions are valid; even if they are valid, it does not guarantee that they are relevant to the daily practice of a particular physician. The history of medicine includes countless examples of therapies that were once widely accepted but were later shown to be ineffective or even harmful to patients. Clinicians must develop skills that will allow them to update and reevaluate their knowledge, enabling them to provide optimal patient care.

SEARCHING THE LITERATURE

The first step in acquiring new medical knowledge is to locate the appropriate literature. This is an increasingly difficult task, as the number of medical journals increases each year. It is not possible for any physician to read, as it is published, everything that is relevant to his or her practice. Fortunately, help of various kinds is available to assist with literature searches, when necessary. In general, the search processes for medical literature include (1) framing the pertinent clinical questions, (2) choosing the literature resources, (3) formulating a search strategy, and (4) deciding on the appropriate literature.

The best online resource to start searching for medical literature is PubMed (http://www.ncbi.nlm.nih.gov/pubmed), a free search engine developed and maintained by the National Library of Medicine, which provides access to MEDLINE, PreMEDLINE,

HealthSTAR, the Cochrane Database of Systematic Reviews, Publisher-Supplied Citations, and other related databases. Other biomedical search engines that one may have access to (depending on personal or institutional subscriptions) include OVID and Embase. In addition, general search engines, such as Google Scholar and Yahoo, have been widely used to gain direct access to the online articles. Because these databases do not overlap entirely, it may be worth searching all of those that one has access to in order to ensure comprehensive coverage. Although the specific methods of searching within each of the databases are different, the basic principles outlined here apply across the board. For simplicity, we will focus on PubMed here.

The search strategy should be based on the main concepts that are being examined. The terms that are used to conduct the literature search should be determined by the study hypothesis, the research questions, and the database in which the search is to be conducted. Moreover, the search should be reproducible. An experienced medical librarian can be invaluable in designing and executing a comprehensive search. The specification of search terms should be thoroughly vetted with the review team to ensure that the appropriate studies are identified and that any systematic bias related to the search criteria is avoided.

The first important search tool to be aware of in PubMed is the Medical Subject Heading (MeSH) browser (http://www.nlm.nih.gov/mesh/meshhome.html). MeSH terms are a detailed taxonomy of keywords that were developed by the National Library of Medicine to cover all the topics in biomedicine. They automatically "explode out" to search for alternate or related terms and spellings so that one does not have to identify and search for each of these separately. Depending on the particular MeSH term that is searched, this feature can cast a very wide net. However, at this point in the search, one wants to be more inclusive than exclusive; it is much easier to discard nonrelevant papers as the review process continues than to identify studies that were missed by too narrow a search. The MeSH browser should be used to identify the relevant MeSH terms for the research question.

MeSH terms do, however, have one important limitation to keep in mind. Because the process of indexing articles and assigning the relevant MeSH terms and characteristics (e.g., language, study type) that can be used to filter the search results takes time, recently published articles that are listed in PubMed may not be captured by a search that relies entirely on MeSH terms. If one is researching a topic that has been receiving a substantial amount of recent attention, one might need to include free-text terms as well as MeSH terms to avoid missing the most recent evidence.

After the search terms are chosen, PubMed allows one to combine them using Boolean connectors (AND, OR, NOT). For more information about searching in PubMed, see the tutorial available online (http://www.nlm.nih.gov/bsd/disted/pubmedtutorial/cover.html). In the example of dietary fat intake and the risk of developing breast cancer, a search like the following might be used: "dietary fats"[MeSH Terms] AND "breast neoplasms"[MeSH Terms] AND risk. This search returns far more results than the articles that will help answer our question; for example, it will capture editorials that do not report any original research results. PubMed provides filtering options that can help reduce the number of unwanted articles one has to sift through. For example, here the search results might be limited to (1) Article types: randomized controlled trial, comparative study, meta-analysis, review, systematic review, multi-center study, OR observational study; (2) Species: humans; (3) Language: English; and (4) Publication dates: a specific time period, which could reduce the number of articles to a reasonable amount. With the advent of computer technology, it has become possible to search the medical literature in an automated manner. For example, a search through a standard database, such as MEDLINE, could be performed to assemble lists of articles that might be of interest. MEDLINE is a database of articles published in any one of almost 4000 biomedical journals. The earliest citations in this database are from 1966, with coverage up through the present time. Although journals from 70 different countries are included in MEDLINE, the vast majority are English language publications. The National Library of Medicine has made the MEDLINE database available through the Internet at the following address: http://www.ncbi.nlm.nih.gov/PubMed.

The search process is based on a few key words that were chosen to recover articles on relevant subjects. The search can be limited to a specific time period, which is helpful if you want to focus on the most recently published information. For example, a recent MEDLINE search for the title words "breast cancer and dietary fat" retrieved approximately 120 journal articles over the previous 2-year period. These articles included a range of investigations, including animal studies, descriptive studies, case-control studies, cohort studies, randomized controlled clinical trials, and reviews, including meta-analyses. Most computer databases include abstracts of the articles from major journals, and some even include the entire text of articles from selected publications.

REVIEWING INDIVIDUAL STUDIES

Once the appropriate literature has been identified, it is useful to apply a uniform and thorough approach to evaluating the articles. This process will encourage the reader to consider all aspects of a study before passing judgment on its validity and utility. The following sections provide one such approach for evaluating individual published studies. The steps in the review are presented in the general sequence in which they should be considered (Table 10-1). Each component of a review is dependent on the others to some extent; however, they are often considered collectively. It is necessary to consider **internal validity**, **clinical importance**, and **external validity** in the critical appraisal of medical studies. The details of the review process for an individual paper are outlined in Table 10-1.

Table 10-1 Stepwise approach to critical appraisal of published medical research.

Internal Validity

Step 1. Consider the research hypothesis
Is there a clear statement on the research hypothesis?
Does the study address a question that has clinical relevance?

Step 2. Consider the study design
Is the study design appropriate for the hypothesis?
Does the design represent an advance over prior approaches?
Does the study use an experimental or an observational design?

Step 3. Consider the outcome variable
Is the outcome being studied relevant to clinical practice?
What criteria are used to define the presence of disease?
Is the determination of the presence or absence of disease accurate?

Step 4. Consider the predictor variable(s)
How many exposures or risk factors are being studied?
How is the presence or absence of exposure determined?
Is the assessment of exposure likely to be precise and accurate?
Is there an attempt to quantify the amount or duration of exposure?
Are biological markers of exposure used in the study?

Step 5. Consider the methods of analysis
Are the employed statistical methods suitable for the types of variables (nominal versus ordinal versus continuous) in the study?
Have the levels of type I and type II errors been discussed appropriately?
Is the sample size adequate to answer the research question?
Have the assumptions underlying the statistical tests been met?
Has chance been evaluated as a potential explanation of the results?

Step 6. Consider the possible sources of bias (systematic errors)
Is the method of selection of subjects likely to have biased results?
Is the measurement of either the exposure or the disease likely to be biased?
Have the investigators considered whether confounders could account for the observed results?
In what direction would each potential bias influence the results?

Clinical Importance

Step 7. Consider the interpretation of results
How large is the observed effect?
Is there evidence of a dose-response relationship?
Are the findings consistent with laboratory models?
Are the effects biologically plausible?
If the findings are negative, was there sufficient statistical power to detect an effect?

External Validity

Step 8. Consider how the results of the study can be used in practice
Are the findings consistent with other studies on the same questions?
Can the findings be generalized to other human populations?
Do the findings warrant a change in current clinical practice?

RESEARCH HYPOTHESIS

It is important to consider the research hypothesis that is being addressed by the study. In practice, this may be a difficult task. Authors often do not state the hypotheses that they wish to test. Sometimes the goal of the study is stated as a research question, but occasionally the reader is left to infer the purpose of the study from a set of complicated analyses.

Once the purpose of the study is discerned, the reader should attempt to determine whether the study addresses a question that has clinical importance. If the study does not, the results may have little relevance to clinical practice. For the physician who needs information to counsel a patient on the relationship between dietary fat and the risk of breast cancer, it is necessary to identify the articles that address that topic. A number of different kinds of hypotheses, however, may be relevant to the general topic. For example, a study on the effects of varying dietary fat composition on the occurrence of mammary tumors in mice may be useful, as studies conducted in laboratory animals can be more tightly controlled than studies conducted in humans. It may be useful to read a study on the effect of a high-fat diet on circulating estrogen levels in women, as this research may be relevant to the biological plausibility of a potential relationship between dietary fat and breast cancer. This type of research may yield information about the mechanism of disease development and prevention.

The various types of **significance** that may be ascribed to a research finding should be distinguished (Table 10-2). It is common to refer to the results as significant if a statistical test indicates that the findings are unlikely to be attributable to chance alone. The evaluation of statistical significance—and therefore the likelihood of committing a type I (false-positive) error—is useful in the interpretation of results.

Even if a finding is statistically significant, however, it may not be biologically or clinically important. For instance, a small difference in the risk of developing breast cancer with increasing levels of dietary fat could be judged to be statistically significant if the finding was based on a large number of observations. Nevertheless, this elevation in risk may be so small that an individual woman's risk of developing breast cancer would not be appreciably altered by changing her diet. As a result, a clinical recommendation to reduce dietary fat might not be supported by the evidence. The biological significance of a finding addresses yet another issue: Do the epidemiologic observations help to clarify the causal mechanism? This type of insight is most likely to be gained if the epidemiologic study involves biological markers of exposure, susceptibility, and outcome.

Table 10-2 Types of significance in clinical research.

Type	Meaning	Assessment
Statistical	Exclusion of chance as an explanation for findings	Statistical test
Clinical	Importance of findings for changing current clinical practice	Magnitude of clinical response to an intervention
Biological	Findings help to clarify the mechanism of action	Compare findings to information from in vitro and in vivo laboratory experimentation

STUDY DESIGN

If the study question is of interest, the reader should then determine what type of study design was employed. As noted in Chapters 4-7, certain designs may be more or less useful in answering specific kinds of questions. Another factor that may have determined the type of study design used by the investigator is the current state of knowledge. Early studies on a particular hypothesis may have a simple design, such as a descriptive study. As the hypothesis is refined, more definitive study designs can be utilized.

The appropriateness of the study design for the research question should be assessed. The incidence rate of the disease in question may be a determining factor. For example, although breast cancer is the most common form of cancer among women in the

United States, this disease is diagnosed among only a small proportion of women during a short period of time. Accordingly, a case-control study would offer an efficient approach to studying this disease, since the sampling scheme for this type of study identifies affected women once they are diagnosed. In fact, studies on dietary fat intake and the occurrence of breast cancer have utilized several different designs, including descriptive, case-control, cohort studies, and clinical trials. Descriptive studies are useful for hypothesis generation, but not for hypothesis testing. The case-control and cohort designs provide more compelling evidence to test specific hypotheses. Randomized controlled trials designs are the optimal solution for the ultimate test of this hypothesis.

OUTCOME VARIABLE

The outcome of interest in the Patient Profile is the development of breast cancer. In investigations of the relationship between dietary fat intake and the risk of developing breast cancer, it is important to specify how the presence or absence of breast cancer was determined. There are several possibilities.

(1) Death certificates limit the information to deceased subjects. In addition, a variety of studies have shown that the information on death certificates may be incomplete or inaccurate.

(2) Self-reports require subjects to be alive or have relatives who can provide information on their breast cancer. If the subjects are not medically sophisticated, they may mistake benign forms of breast disease for breast cancer.

(3) Medical records may provide more accurate information than death certificates or self-reports. However, it is possible that the diagnostic criteria differ from physician to physician, over time, or across geographic regions or countries.

(4) Histopathologic diagnoses provide the most definitive information, but adequate tissue must be available for pathologic examination.

It is desirable to have the most definitive information possible on the presence of disease. This will tend to minimize the likelihood of the misclassification of subjects. For breast cancer, it is possible that

a small proportion of apparently health women may actually have occult (undiscovered) breast cancer. This could be evaluated by performing a screening test, such as mammography, on all apparently unaffected subjects. Because so few asymptomatic cancers are likely to be detected, however, the study findings would probably not be greatly affected by limiting the detection to routine histopathologic diagnosis.

It is also important to judge how precisely the investigator defines the outcome. In general, it is useful to specify a single disease entity when searching for causes. For example, a study of dietary fat and the risk of all cancers combined may produce misleading results, as different cancers have different causes, and only some causes may involve dietary fat. Restricting the study to breast cancer improves the likelihood of obtaining a definitive result for this disease of primary interest.

PREDICTOR VARIABLES

The predictor variable is the risk factor or exposure under investigation. Studies may involve a single risk factor of interest or several different predictor variables. If a number of exposure variables are included, they may not be closely linked.

In a study on the cause of breast cancer, an investigator might choose to examine a variety of exposure variables, including reproductive factors, such as age at first full-term pregnancy, hormone levels, exposure to radiation, and dietary fat intake. Although this sort of study may provide a more comprehensive picture of the cause of breast cancer, it may limit the ability to collect detailed information on each exposure of interest. Even if a study is focused on the question of dietary fat and the risk of developing breast cancer, it is necessary to collect some basic information on other possible determinants of breast cancer that could act as confounders.

The reader must determine whether the methods used to characterize the presence or absence of exposure are reliable and accurate. Possible methods of ascertainment include subject or surrogate respondent reports, direct observation, or measurement of a biological marker. The reader should ask whether there are better ways to define the exposure levels of subjects.

The assessment of a dietary exposure can be particularly difficult. In one method, subjects are asked about their past dietary habits and must remember the kinds and the amounts of foods that they ate. Various studies have indicated that such recall, although imperfect, may suffice for determining whether a subject consumed a relatively high, moderate, or low amount of dietary fat. Generally, it is desirable to have several levels of exposure defined so that a dose-response relationship can be evaluated.

Another approach to determining dietary fat intake is to have subjects record what they currently eat. This can be done by keeping a diary or by using a list of commonly eaten foods to check off the meals and snacks that are being ingested. There are problems with this approach, however. Subjects may forget to record what they eat, or they may incorrectly estimate the size of portions. To help offset such problems, plastic models of different portion sizes are available to provide visual cues and reminders. It is important to remember that a subject's current diet may not accurately reflect his past diet. In a case-control design based only on current diet information, it is crucial to know whether the subjects with breast cancer changed their diets because of (1) the disease, (2) the side effects of treatment, or (3) the hope of influencing prognosis.

Another approach to collecting information on diet is to measure what subjects eat; this approach could be useful for a prospective cohort study in which the subjects are followed to determine whether they develop breast cancer. This approach to measuring dietary intake would be extremely difficult in practice, however, as it would require a tightly controlled environment in which the investigator could observe the foods eaten by subjects.

Epidemiologists occasionally take advantage of a situation in which people maintain certain dietary habits for religious or other reasons. Thus, an epidemiologist may identify a group of people (e.g., vegetarians) who consume very little fat in their diets. The frequency of occurrence of breast cancer in this group could be compared with the experience of another group whose members consume large amounts of fat. The problem of determining the precise intake of fat for subjects in each group remains, however. Furthermore, it is likely that the groups will differ in lifestyle factors other than the intake of dietary fat, giving rise to potential confounding.

The use of biological markers of exposure has become more common in clinical research. Biological markers are important because they can provide quantitative documentation of exposure in certain circumstances. No biological markers of fat intake are currently available, but to assess the long-term intake of dietary fat, the fatty acid content of adipose tissue could be measured in biopsies. Obviously, the utility of such a measure depends on the extent to which it accurately reflects consumption patterns. The willingness of study participants to undergo a tissue biopsy must also be considered.

METHODS OF ANALYSIS

The emphasis placed on a particular research finding often depends on the ability of the investigator to exclude chance as an explanation for the observed results. This is accomplished by the use of statistical tests. Readers should have a basic understanding of which statistical tests are appropriate for which types of analysis. The type of statistical test that should be used is determined by the goal of the analysis (e.g., to compare groups, to explore an association, or to predict an outcome) and the types of variables used in the analysis (e.g., categorical, ordinal, or continuous variables).

By convention, the 5% level of statistical significance is used as a standard in many biomedical studies. That is, the investigator is willing to accept a 1 in 20 risk that the observed effect is a result of chance variation alone. Care must be taken to avoid oversimplistic interpretations of P-values, however. One common mistake is to assume that a statistically significant result is biologically or clinically important. As discussed above, the clinical importance and biological plausibility of the results are not assessed by the hypothesis tests.

A second common mistake is to dismiss a finding because it has not reached the predetermined level of statistical significance. A P-value of 0.08, for example, although not statistically significant in common practice, still represents a finding that is relatively unlikely to be attributable to chance. It would be unwise, therefore, to conclude on the basis of such a P-value that there is no relationship between dietary fat intake and the development of breast cancer in a particular study. A heavy reliance on P-values is particularly dangerous when the sample size of a study is small and the statistical power is therefore low as well. In such situations, even moderate differences between groups may fail to reach a conventional level of statistical significance, and the ability to reach a definitive conclusion is limited.

POSSIBLE SOURCES OF BIAS

A result must also be examined to determine whether it could be due to systematic errors that are related to the sampling strategy or to data collection procedures. A statistical test cannot address whether biases of any sort are responsible for the observed results. As discussed in Chapter 9, the consideration of potential bias often cannot be assessed in precise quantitative terms. Bias can occur in any study, although certain designs are more susceptible to specific types of bias. Regardless of the study design, the potential for three distinct types of bias should be considered (Table 10-3).

Table 10-3 Types of bias in clinical research.

Bias	Source of Error
Selection bias	Sample distorted by the selection process
Information bias	Misclassification of the variables
Confounding	An extraneous variable that accounts for the observed result rather than the risk factor of interest

The first concern is whether the selection of subjects is likely to have distorted the results (**selection bias**). Because few studies (if any) can examine an entire population, the investigator must draw a sample to make inferences about the population.

The reader must determine whether the samples are likely to be representative of the population to which extrapolations are made.

The methods section of any published medical research paper should include details on how the subjects were selected for the study. In a case-control study, a selection bias could arise from the approach used to select cases, controls, or both. In the context of a case-control study on dietary fat and the occurrence of breast cancer, a selection bias might occur if prevalent (surviving) cases are used rather than newly diagnosed (incident) cases. This distortion would occur if the prediagnostic nutritional status were related to disease prognosis. For example, if women who consumed high-fat diets before developing breast cancer survived longer than women who consumed low-fat diets, the prevalent cases would overrepresent high-fat consumption, and the observed risk ratio may be biased toward large values. The bias is presented schematically in Figure 10-1.

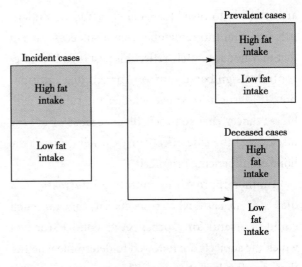

Figure 10-1. Schematic diagram of the bias introduced by a study of prevalent cases when the risk factor (high fat intake) is related to the prognosis. The shaded areas represent cases with high fat intake and the unshaded areas represent cases with low fat intake. Note that the deceased cases included a relatively large proportion of persons with diets low in fat, resulting in an overrepresentation of the high-fat consumers among the prevalent cases.

In a case-control study, the sampling of controls can be as great of a source of selection bias as the sampling of cases. Consider a hospital-based sample of control subjects with diagnoses other than breast cancer. If the diseases of the control subjects are caused by dietary factors (e.g., atherosclerotic heart disease) or, conversely, if the diseases influence dietary intake (e.g., gastrointestinal disease), a biased case-control comparison may result. Sampling from the general population typically results in control subjects who better reflect the exposure patterns of persons without the disease of interest. Even general population sampling schemes can result in a distorted control group, however. For example, a telephone sampling technique might preferentially include higher income women, as they are more likely to have telephones than lower income women. Additionally, if higher income women are less likely to work outside of the home, they would be more available when the sampling is performed. Because the diets of higher income women may differ from those of other women, a biased case-control comparison may occur. To determine whether a telephone sampling scheme is likely to yield an unbiased sample of control subjects, it is necessary to know the completeness of telephone coverage in the target population. Additionally, multiple calls should be made to the sampled residences at varying times of the day and days of the week to reach persons who work outside the home.

Cohort studies on the association between dietary factors and the occurrence of breast cancer are also subject to a potential selection bias. The major source of selection bias in such studies is a loss to follow-up during the study. If women who eat a high-fat diet and develop breast cancer tend to discontinue participation in the study for some reason prior to the diagnosis of cancer, the investigator will underestimate the risk of developing breast cancer in women whose diets are high in fat. To date, cohort studies of this question have yielded conflicting results. An important consideration in such a situation is the extent to which the bias due to loss in follow-up can explain the discrepancy.

Another source of bias can arise from systematic errors in measuring either the independent variable (exposure) or the dependent variable (disease). This type of bias is often referred to as **information bias** or **misclassification bias**. For example, in a case-control study, the validity of the information on exposure may be questioned because the data are gathered retrospectively. Because the cases are aware of their disease and have undergone treatment for it, their reporting of past exposures may differ systematically from the reporting of control subjects. This is referred to as **recall bias**. Studies on dietary risk factors may be susceptible to recall bias. For example, if patients with breast cancer have wondered why they developed their cancer, they may tend to overestimate past exposure to dietary fat, particularly when the potential relationship has been widely publicized. Control subjects may be less concerned about their past diet or may be worried about other problems, such as obesity, which would tend to make them underreport their exposure to dietary fat.

If recall bias occurred in a study, the investigator might overestimate the relationship between dietary fat intake and the risk of developing breast cancer. In fact, a number of studies have demonstrated problems of imperfect recall in dietary history. Only a few studies, however, have examined differential (biased) recall in cases versus controls by comparing prospectively collected dietary data with subsequent data that was retrospectively collected from the same subjects. In general, these investigations have not demonstrated a differential recall of food intake in cases of breast cancer compared with the controls. This would suggest that recall bias is an unlikely explanation for the inconsistent results that are reported from case-control studies on the association of dietary fat intake and the occurrence of breast cancer.

It should be remembered, however, that even if cases and controls do not differ in the ability to recall dietary exposure, misclassification bias could still occur. Errors in reporting that are comparable between the cases and controls give rise to nondifferential misclassification. If nondifferential misclassification occurs, it may reduce the estimated risk ratio. In other words, such misclassification tends to make it more difficult to detect any true differences between the cases and controls.

The final consideration of bias is to determine whether **confounding** can account for the observed results. A confounder is an extraneous correlate of disease that, because of its association with the risk factor of interest, accounts for some or all of the observed association between the risk factor and the disease. In studies of dietary fat intake and the occurrence of breast cancer, it is important to determine whether the investigator has accounted for the effects of known risk factors for breast cancer. These factors include age, race, reproductive characteristics (e.g., age at first full-term pregnancy, number of pregnancies, duration of lactation), obesity among post-menopausal women, alcohol intake, and exposure to radiation. A schematic diagram for confounding of the relationship between dietary fat intake and the occurrence of breast cancer by the number of pregnancies is presented in Figure 10-2. If women who eat a high-fat diet have fewer pregnancies than those who eat a low-fat diet, an apparent association between the consumption of dietary fat and the occurrence of breast cancer could be attributable to the effects of reproductive history rather than those of diet, per se.

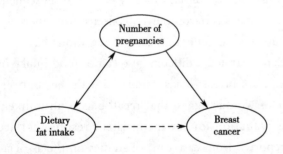

Figure 10-2. Schematic diagram of confounding of the dietary fat-breast cancer relationship by the number of pregnancies.

In an observational study, confounding can be controlled either in the design of the study (by restricting subject inclusion to persons with a narrow range of the confounder values or by matching study groups to confounders) or in the analysis of the results (through stratification by confounders or by regression techniques). All of these adjustment methods, however, are contingent on knowing which variables are confounders. Because the known risk factors for developing breast cancer do not account for all occurrences of the disease, other unknown risk factors must exist. Any observed association between dietary fat intake and the occurrence of breast cancer could be explained, at least in part, in that way.

When the reader detects a potential for bias, it is important to try to estimate both the magnitude and the direction of the effect that the bias could have on the results. In this way, the reader can determine if the bias is likely to have inflated the results or to have diminished the exposure's effect. In a case-control study, for example, if it is suspected that women with breast cancer are more likely than control subjects to remember and report fat intake, the risk ratio could be overestimated. In contrast, if it seems likely that patients with breast cancer underreport their dietary fat intake in comparison to the control subjects, the observed results may underestimate the true impact of dietary fat intake on the occurrence of breast cancer. In discussing the results, an investigator may attempt to convince the reader that the magnitude of bias would not be sufficient to skew the results, or that the true relationship is as strong as or stronger than that observed.

INTERPRETATION OF RESULTS

If the investigator reports a statistically significant result that cannot be explained by bias, the reader must then decide whether the result is clinically important. Consider, for example, a study concluding that a 50% decrease in dietary fat intake is associated with a 5% decrease in the risk of developing breast cancer. Even if this result is statistically significant, the magnitude of the reduction in risk is so slight in exchange for the major change required in diet that individual patients may be poorly motivated to make the dietary change. On the other hand, the benefit to society in eliminating 5% of all breast cancer cases may well justify a mass public education effort to reduce the consumption of dietary fat.

Conversely, results that are not statistically significant need not be considered useless. In particular, when there is a small sample size or when the relationship between the exposure and the disease is weak, the possibility of a false-negative conclusion must be considered. The statistical power of the study to detect the observed effect may be too low to allow for a definitive conclusion from the study.

PRACTICAL UTILITY OF RESULTS

When reviewing a published study, the reader must determine the practical utility of the results. The usefulness of a study finding depends on various factors, including the purpose of the study, the limitations of the study population, the clinical and biological importance of the results, and the study's consistency with findings from other published studies. Clinical and epidemiologic research have various purposes. The clinical utility of a particular research finding must be viewed in the context of the type of question that is posed. As indicated in Table 10-4, a particular study may lead to findings that are relevant to disease causation, early detection of the disease, the prediction of prognosis, or improved treatment. Studies on the relationship between dietary fat intake and the occurrence of breast cancer relate to disease causation. Unfortunately, there is no standard by which to judge whether an association between a risk factor and a disease is clinically important. Clearly, the stronger the association (i.e., the farther the risk ratio is from the null value), the greater the potential impact of eliminating the exposure. In assessing clinical utility, consideration must be given to how difficult it is to change the risk factor (in this case, to reduce dietary fat intake) and to the amount of morbidity and mortality associated with the disease.

Table 10-4   Clinical applications of various types of studies.

Type of Study	Application to Clinical Practice
Etiologic	Can risk be reduced among susceptible persons?
Diagnostic	Can accuracy and timeliness or diagnosis be improved?
Prognostic	Can prognosis be determined more definitively?
Therapeutic	Can treatment be improved?

The ability to generalize the findings beyond the study population should be taken into account.

For this purpose, the definition and limitations of the study sample must be understood. For example, some studies of risk factors for developing breast cancer have focused on postmenopausal women. This may limit the applicability of such studies to the premenopausal patient in the Patient Profile. Investigators are often forced to restrict the sample by age, race, or other factors. The reader must decide what effect these restrictions may have on the broader applicability of results.

In determining whether the findings of a particular study can be generalized to other populations, it is useful to assess whether similar results have been obtained in other studies. It often occurs that the first evaluation of a risk factor, diagnostic test, or therapeutic regimen is favorable, whereas subsequent reports demonstrate more limited utility. One reason for this pattern is that initial assessments often involve selected populations that offer a best-case scenario. Subsequent attempts to broaden the applicability may prove to be less successful.

ESTABLISHING A CAUSAL RELATIONSHIP

Ultimately, the reader may question whether a causal relationship between a risk factor and the occurrence of a disease has been supported by the results of a study. Table 10-5 presents selected criteria that can be used to evaluate suspected causal relationships. The consideration of causality is based on the findings of a particular study within the context of what is already known about a disease process.

Table 10-5   Selected criteria for evaluating a suspected causal relationship.

Strength
Presence of a dose-response relationship
Correct temporal sequence
Consistency of results across studies
Biological plausibility

The **strength of observed association** is a primary criterion in evaluating whether a risk factor causes a disease. The strength of the association is indicated by the distance of the risk ratio or odds ratio from the null value. When the association is very strong, it is less likely that the association can be explained by chance or bias. Weak associations also may be causal, indicating only a lower risk of disease development. With a weak association, however, it is more difficult to exclude other factors and biases that may account for the relationship.

It is useful to examine whether there is a **dose-response relationship** between the proposed risk factor and the disease. If there is, increased levels of the risk factor will be associated with a greater risk of developing the disease (or with protection in the case of a beneficial factor). For example, as the level of dietary fat intake increases, the risk of developing breast cancer would be expected to increase if a causal relationship exists (Figure 10-3). The absence of a progressive, graded dose-response relationship does not preclude a causal relationship, however. For example, there may be a threshold above which the level of the risk factor confers increased risk. In this case, the risk of disease will not be affected by changes in exposure below a certain level, but the risk does vary with exposure at higher levels.

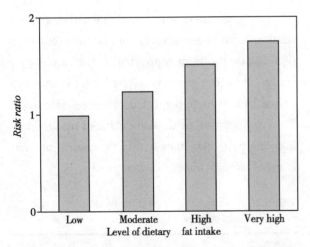

Figure 10-3. Hypothetical dose-response relationship between the level of dietary fat intake and the risk ratio of developing breast cancer. The reference category of exposure is low dietary fat intake.

With any association, it is helpful to compare the findings with the results of other studies. If other investigators studying different populations in differing settings find similar results, a causal explanation is supported. However, the reader must be careful when judging the consistency of the results, as it is possible that the same flaw could lead to incorrect conclusions in several studies.

The proposed causal relationship should be consistent with what is currently known about biology and the disease process. This is often referred to as **biological plausibility**. If the proposed cause-and-effect relationship is not in accordance with current knowledge, the causality may be questioned. The assessment of biological plausibility often requires a review of research on other human populations, as well as a review of research that involves laboratory animal models.

The **temporal relationship** between a suspected cause and an effect is important. That is, *a cause must always precede an effect in time*. This seems intuitive, but, in reality, factors that are suspected to be causes sometimes turn out to be effects of the disease. For example, a person with an early undiagnosed cancer may make a change in food choices because of the unrecognized systemic effects of the cancer. Consequently, the dietary change may appear to be the cause of, rather than an effect of, the later diagnosed cancer. Case-control studies of chronic diseases with long latent periods are particularly susceptible to this problem. For a factor to be considered the cause of a disease, it is theoretically important that the removal or modification of that factor will prevent the disease from occurring or will ameliorate the disease once it has occurred.

In practice, the criterion of removal or modification of a suspected causal factor may not always be satisfied. There are some instances in which a causal factor may set off a protracted chain of events. Once established, this sequence may no longer depend on the presence of the causal agent for progression. For example, many cancers are thought to develop in response to an initiating event, followed by promotional effects that occur for many years. If the risk factor of interest contributes to initiation only, removal of the exposure during the promotional phase will not affect the subsequent risk of developing cancer. Thus, eliminating an initiating risk factor for cancer may not affect the incidence of this disease for many years into the future.

DIETARY FAT AND BREAST CANCER

As mentioned previously, the relationship between dietary fat intake and the risk of developing breast cancer was investigated in a variety of epidemiologic studies. These studies included case series reports, ecologic analyses, case-control studies, cohort studies, clinical trials, and systematic reviews.

OBSERVATIONAL STUDIES

Ecologic or correlation studies have demonstrated a consistently strong relationship between dietary habits, as estimated by the per-capita consumption of dietary fat, and breast cancer occurrence in different countries. Plots of these data have yielded a linear relationship, with increasing fat consumption associated with higher breast cancer occurrence. The problem with such studies is that they do not demonstrate that increased dietary fat in *individuals* is associated with breast cancer occurrence in the same individuals (i.e., an **ecological fallacy** may be involved). For example, in industrialized countries, fat consumption and breast cancer mortality tend to be higher than in developing countries; however, it may not be the high fat consumers who are developing breast cancer in industrialized countries. The comparatively high mortality rates of breast cancer in industrialized countries may be attributable to other factors, such as earlier menarche, delayed childbearing, or other reproductive factors.

Case-control studies have yielded conflicting results on the question of diet and breast cancer. The reasons for these conflicting results are not clear. One criticism is that dietary data that are collected retrospectively are inaccurate (i.e., dietary exposure is misclassified). General difficulties in recalling diet could contribute to nondifferential misclassification, and case-control differences in the ability or motivation to recall dietary fat could result in differential misclassification. Another potential explanation is that the influence of dietary fat could have been exerted many years prior to the diagnosis of breast cancer. Most case-control studies have included diet information from the recent past, but not from the remote past. Some reviewers have concluded that none of the studies, when viewed individually, had a large enough sample size to provide adequate statistical power. In other words, a true relationship between dietary fat intake and the risk of developing breast cancer might be missed because of inadequate discriminatory ability (i.e., a type II error may be involved).

Some of these problems can be avoided with a cohort study design. Prospective cohort studies eliminate the potential for distortion of the results from a differential recall of dietary history. This type of study was used to investigate the question of fat in the diet and the risk of developing breast cancer. Again, the published results of cohort studies on this question have yielded conflicting results. Some studies have produced evidence of a relatively weak association, with risk ratios of approximately 1.4. Other cohort studies, however, have actually indicated that increased dietary fat intake may protect against the development of breast cancer. The Nurses' Health Study was a cohort study of 88,795 women who were free of cancer in 1980 and were then followed for the subsequent development of cancer. Through 14 years of follow-up, a total of 2,965 women were diagnosed with breast cancer. In this population, no association was observed between a reduced intake of total fat, or major subtypes of fat, and the risk of developing breast cancer.

In general, the dose-response relationship suggested by the ecologic studies has not been borne out in the case-control and cohort studies. Some reviewers have argued that the range of dietary fat intake in the analytic studies is smaller than in the international ecologic studies. Within a single country, there may be too little variation in fat intake to demonstrate a dose-response relationship in case-control and cohort studies. Others have argued that factors other than diet (i.e., confounders) that could not be easily controlled in ecologic studies were the real explanation for the association between fat intake and the development of breast cancer that was observed in the correlation analyses.

CLINICAL TRIALS

A large, randomized, controlled trial is the best way to resolve the issue of the relationship between dietary fat intake and the risk of developing breast cancer. To date, 3 randomized controlled trials have consistently reported that a low-fat diet did not significantly reduce the risk of breast cancer. The Women's Health Initiative randomized low-fat dietary modification trial was conducted in 40 U.S. clinical centers from 1993 to 2005. A total of 48,835 postmenopausal women without prior breast cancer were enrolled. Over an 8.1-year average follow-up period, the hazard ratio comparing the low-fat diet group with the usual diet group was 0.91 (95% confidence interval: 0.83 to 1.01) for invasive breast cancer. Clearly, this type of study would provide the most definitive evidence about a causal relationship between the consumption of dietary fat and the risk of developing breast cancer. This is mainly owing to the principal strength of clinical trial designs (compared to observational studies), which derives from assigning treatments to subjects by **randomization**, thereby tending to balance the study groups with respect to both known and unknown confounders. The current trials, however, are slightly limited for excluding the potential influence of any lifestyle changes that result from adopting a low-fat dietary pattern.

MECHANISTIC STUDIES

Was there biological plausibility to the relationship? What pathophysiologic mechanism might be involved? Were there animal models that showed the relationship between fat in the diet and the development of breast cancer? In fact, animal studies have found an association between fat intake and the development of mammary cancers in mice bearing the mammary tumor virus. Similar findings have been reported in other animal models. The pathophysiology involved in this process is less clear, but potential mechanisms have been discussed. It has been speculated that mammary neoplasms are controlled by an endocrine balance, which in turn is affected by dietary factors, including fat intake. For example, women consuming high-fat diets have been shown to have more circulating estrogen than women on low-fat diets. In postmenopausal women, adipose tissue has been demonstrated to be a contributor to the production of estrogen. Dietary fat intake may also have modified DNA synthesis and cell duplication. If this were found to be true for breast tissue, this could be relevant to breast carcinogenesis. In animal studies, certain types of fatty acids in the diet modulate mammary tumor growth and metastasis. The evidence is strongest for the promotional effect of polyunsaturated fat. The potential differential effect of various types of fatty acids on the development and progression of cancer might explain some of the variation observed in the studies of fat intake and breast cancer risk in humans. Most epidemiologic studies have evaluated total fat intake. Some studies have used the adipose tissue levels of fat as a surrogate for the measurement of fat intake. Adipose tissue levels, however, do not provide an indication of the dietary intake of fatty acids that can be synthesized internally. The Nurses' Health Study did include a prospective evaluation of the different types of fatty acid intake. In this study, none of the various types of dietary fat was associated with the risk of developing breast cancer.

SYSTEMATIC REVIEWS

A **systematic review** is any type of synthesis of evidence on a topic that has been prepared using strategies to minimize errors. A **meta-analysis** is a type of quantitative systematic review in which the results of multiple studies that are considered combinable are aggregated together to obtain a precise, and hopefully unbiased, estimate of the relationship in question. As already illustrated in the dietary fat-breast cancer question, single studies rarely provide a definitive answer on a topic. A systematic review helps in two specific ways:

(1) By combining a series of smaller studies, each

with a statistically imprecise estimate of effect, a larger sample size is obtained, with a corresponding increase in statistical precision.

(2) By identifying the differences in findings across different studies, sensitivity analyses can be conducted, which may lead to greater insight into the sources of heterogeneity.

The steps in a systematic review should follow a clear sequence. We will introduce the systematic review in detail in Chapter 11. In the context of the Patient Profile, we might specify the question in the following way: *For premenopausal women with a family history of breast cancer, is the reduction of dietary fat consumption substantially below the typical levels in the American diet likely to reduce the risk of developing breast cancer?* Here, for simplicity, we briefly explain the pooled estimate of effect size for multiple studies with a hypothetical meta-analysis.

The actual analysis of the data begins with an estimation of the effect of interest in each of the included studies. It is useful to display the individual study results as shown in Figure 10-4. In this graph, the results of five separate hypothetical studies on the relationship between reduced dietary fat intake and the risk of developing breast cancer are presented. The findings of each investigation are summarized with a point estimate of the effect and a corresponding confidence interval around that estimate. The point estimate is represented as a solid circle, with a horizontal line stretching in both directions to the upper and lower bounds of the confidence interval. By convention, the effect typically is measured in terms of either an odds ratio or a relative risk (risk ratio).

In Figure 10-4, the results are displayed in terms of an estimated relative risk of developing breast cancer that is associated with a reduced level of dietary fat intake. If reducing fat in the diet decreases the risk of developing breast cancer, a relative risk less than one would be expected. The point estimates for the relative risks in these hypothetical studies ranged from a low of 0.6 (Study E) to a high of 1.3 (Study A). Four of the five studies (Studies B through E) had point estimates lower than one, which is consistent

with the possibility of a reduction in breast cancer risk. On the other hand, most of these estimates are close to the null value of one (no association between dietary fat intake and the risk of developing breast cancer). It is possible, therefore, that these small benefits suggested by a reduction in fat consumption may have arisen by chance.

Examination of the corresponding confidence intervals for the individual studies provides some insight into the statistical precision of the results and whether they are statistically significant. By convention, 95% confidence limits are typically calculated. The odds or risk ratio is often displayed on a logarithmic scale, as in Figure 10-4, to make the confidence intervals symmetrical around the point estimate.

It can be seen from Figure 10-4 that the precision of the five study results varied, with the narrowest confidence intervals (greatest precision) for Study D and the widest confidence intervals (least precision) for Study A. Only one of the five studies had a result that was statistically significant at the 5% level, as indicated by the fact that its confidence interval did not cross the dashed vertical line corresponding to the null value of one.

Statistical integration of the results of the individual studies allows for calculation of a summary estimate of the effect. On the bottom of Figure 10-4, the combined point estimate for the five hypothetical studies is shown as a diamond. The vertical points of the diamond are located at the point estimate of the summary effect, and the horizontal points are located at the upper and lower bounds of the 95% confidence interval, respectively. In this example, the combined point estimate was 0.86, with a corresponding 95% confidence interval from 0.70 to 1.05. The summary estimate is based on a larger sample size than any of the individual study results. Accordingly, the combined estimate is more precise, which is reflected in the figure by comparatively narrow confidence intervals. In this example, it can be seen that the combined effect is consistent with a small reduction in the risk of developing breast cancer, but even with the large sample size of the five studies combined, chance cannot be excluded as a possible cause of the findings.

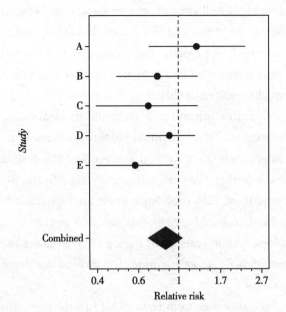

Figure 10-4. Meta-analysis of five hypothetical epidemiologic studies (A-E) on the relationship between reduced dietary fat intake and the risk of developing breast cancer.

Meta-analysis can be useful in achieving greater statistical power, but it cannot overcome the limitations and potential biases of the individual studies. A meta-analysis of case-control studies supported the presence of an association between the increased intake of dietary fat and an elevated risk of developing breast cancer. This systematic review has been criticized, however, on the grounds that the heterogeneity across individual study results was not adequately considered. The investigator performing a meta-analysis must also be careful that the selection of some studies and the exclusion of others do not lead to a distorted conclusion. One meta-analysis on studies of diet and breast cancer combined the results from 12 case-control studies. No relationship between dietary fat intake and the risk of developing breast cancer was found in premenopausal women, but an association between increased fat intake and the risk of developing breast cancer was detected in postmenopausal women with a risk ratio of 1.5. In a statistically combined analysis of 7 international cohorts with an aggregate total of nearly 5,000 cases of breast cancer, the risk ratio for the highest quintile compared to the lowest quintile of total fat intake

was 1.05, with a 95% confidence interval from 0.94 to 1.16. A new meta-analysis of 24 cohort studies, including 38,262 cases, also indicated no significant association of dietary total fat intake with the risk of breast cancer. Thus, the combined result was consistent with little or no elevation in the risk of developing breast cancer in association with an increased intake of fat. Any apparent effect was so small that, even with the considerable sample size of these aggregated studies, chance could not be excluded as a possible explanation for any observed increased risk.

SUGGESTION

In the Patient Profile, the physician wanted to determine whether dietary fat intake is causally related to the development of breast cancer. The findings of the studies were inconsistent, and the strength of the association was modest at best, without clear evidence of a dose-response relationship. The temporal sequence of dietary fat intake and the development of breast cancer appeared to be reasonable.

The physician in the Patient Profile is left with uncertain conclusions from the observational studies and firm evidence from the randomized controlled trials for the question about the relationship between the consumption of dietary fat and the risk of developing breast cancer. Obviously, the evidence in the clinical trials is a prior consideration for an answer to the question about the relationship between the consumption of dietary fat and the risk of developing breast cancer. Even if observational research had demonstrated a small increase in risk with high-fat diets for postmenopausal women, the patient is premenopausal, so it is not clear that the results can be applied to this patient. From another perspective, however, the patient's dietary habits would presumably be continued and could be protective in later life. The physician may also believe that a low-fat diet or dietary fat modification is justifiable for other reasons, including a reduction in the risk for cardiovascular disease. In addition, there are other cancers, such as colon cancer, for which the protective effect of a low-fat diet has been demonstrated more clearly.

This type of uncertainty is common in clinical

medicine. Physicians must often weigh the potential risks and benefits of an intervention and make decisions without complete information. The goal of medical research is to continue to provide more comprehensive answers to important clinical questions.

Much of the satisfaction derived from patient care relates to the ability to incorporate new knowledge into the practice of medicine. It is imperative to develop the skills that are required for a critical review of the medical literature to keep current on the state of information. This is a difficult task, but the reward is enormous when it results in improved patient care.

SUMMARY

In this chapter, a structured approach to reviewing published epidemiologic studies was presented. The ultimate goal of this approach is to help integrate epidemiologic information into clinical practice. As a focus for discussion, the literature on dietary fat intake and the risk of developing breast cancer is used to illustrate the evaluation process.

The initial step in reviewing the medical literature is to conduct a thorough search for relevant recent publications. Screening for appropriate articles can be accomplished through a manual or a computer-assisted approach. In either case, the correct choice of search terms that are calculated to retrieve pertinent articles is essential. Computer searches can save time and, consequently, are extremely popular.

The actual review of a publication begins with the stated purpose of the investigation. For the medical practitioner, a primary consideration is whether a particular study addresses a clinically important question. Are the results likely to influence the delivery of patient care? In the present context, the clinical importance might be assessed in terms of whether the findings support a recommendation to lower dietary fat intake to reduce the risk of developing breast cancer.

The design of an investigation determines the types of inferences that can be drawn from it. The most compelling evidence for cause-and-effect relationships is derived from randomized controlled clinical trials. Among observational investigations, prospective cohort studies are generally the least susceptible to bias, followed by retrospective cohort and case-control studies. Descriptive studies are useful for generating research questions, but not for testing hypotheses.

The measurement of outcome (i.e., development of disease) as well as the documentation of exposure to risk factors can be complicated in observational research. Emphasis must be placed on obtaining the most accurate information possible, recognizing that the ideal often cannot be achieved. Whenever possible, assessment should be performed in a blinded manner and should be based on objective, standard criteria.

A distinction must be made between the concept of statistical significance, which can be evaluated by a hypothesis test, and clinical or biological significance. P-values should not be used to indicate the importance of a finding, but rather, the likelihood that sampling variability can explain the results. Clinical importance relates to whether a difference in outcomes that is observed between the study groups is large enough to warrant a change in clinical practice. Biological significance refers to the extent to which findings help to elucidate the underlying biological processes.

Systematic errors may arise in observational research from the approach to sample selection, information collection, or confounding. It is usually impossible to determine whether a particular bias has actually occurred. Attention, therefore, is focused on strategies to minimize the likelihood that systematic errors will affect the study conclusions. When bias is suspected in an investigation, the exact level of distortion is generally unknown. The direction of the systematic error (i.e., a tendency to either overestimate or underestimate the strength of association) may be clear, however. The assessment of whether an observed association is likely to be one of cause and effect is based on specific criteria, including the strength of association, presence of a dose-response relationship, appropriateness of the temporal sequence of exposure and outcome, consistency of results across studies, and biological plausibility.

When applied to the literature on dietary fat and breast cancer, this process of reasoning leads to an inconclusive assessment. Although consistent supporting evidence comes from the most compelling type of studies (i.e., randomized controlled trial), whether the evidence can be generalized to a specific patient still needs to be assessed. For other studies, in situations in which an association has been observed, the magnitude has generally been weak. The results have been inconsistent across studies, perhaps due in part to limitations in the study design and in part to the weakness of the relationship, even if it exists.

As with many issues in medicine, the dietary fat-breast cancer hypothesis remains cautious. Because little harm probably results from the restriction of dietary fat intake and because other benefits may accrue (i.e., a reduction in the risk of cardiovascular disease), it may be reasonable for the clinician in the Patient Profile to recommend this change in dietary habits to the patient. Until more definitive information is available, however, the patient should be counseled that the effect of restricting dietary fat intake on the risk of developing breast cancer is nonsignificant.

(Qiuan Zhong)

IMPORTANT TERMINOLOGY

medical subject headings	医学主题词表
internal validity	内在真实性
clinical importance	临床重要性
external validity	外在真实性
statistical significance	统计学意义
biological plausibility	生物学合理性
biological marker	生物标志物
systematic error	系统误差
bias	偏倚
nondifferential misclassification	非差异性错误分类
differential misclassification	差异性错误分类
causal relationship	因果关联
strength of association	关联强度
dose-response relationship	剂量 - 反应关系

temporal relationship	关联时序
randomization	随机化
systematic review	系统评价
meta-analysis	荟萃分析

STUDY QUESTIONS

1. *What are the specific approaches to the critical appraisal of published medical research?*

2. *In a cohort study of dietary fat intake and the occurrence of breast cancer, 45% of the subjects are lost to follow up after 2 years. Which of the following bias is most likely to occur?*
   A. *Selection bias*
   B. *Random error*
   C. *Information bias*
   D. *Confounding*

3. *The treatment of mild hypertension is studied in 500 patients who are randomly assigned to either a new antihypertensive medication or a diuretic. Which of the following is the most appropriate study design for assessing this treatment?*
   A. *Case-control study*
   B. *Cohort study*
   C. *Clinical trial*
   D. *Cross-sectional study (descriptive)*

4. *The national prevalence of immunization against hepatitis B was examined in several countries and was found to be inversely associated with the national mortality rates for liver cancer. The most appropriate study design for this research is*
   A. *Case-control study*
   B. *Cohort study*
   C. *Cross-sectional study (descriptive)*
   D. *Ecologic study*

5. *In a cohort study on the relationship between left ventricular mass, as determined by echocardiography, and the incidence of myocardial infarction, it was found that, relative to normal left ventricular mass, the relative risks were 1.5 for mild elevation (95% confidence interval, CI: 1.0 to 2.2), 1.9 for moderate elevation (95% CI: 1.4 to 2.4), and 3.0 for severe elevation (95% CI: 2.1 to 4.3). For this situation, the most appropriate criteria for establishing a causal relationship refers to*

A. *Strength of association*

B. *Dose-response relationship*

C. *Correct temporal sequence*

D. *Consistency of results*

FURTHER READING

McTiernan A, Gilligan MA, Redmond C: Assessing individual risk for breast cancer: Risky business. *J Clin Epidemiol.* 1997;50:547-556.

Kushi L, Giovannucci E: Dietary fat and cancer. *Am J Med.* 2002;113(Suppl):S63-70.

U.S. National Library of Medicine: PubMed.gov. http://www.ncbi.nlm.nih.gov/pubmed.

REFERENCES

Critical Review

Steinbrook R. Searching for the right search---reaching the medical literature. *N Engl J Med.* 2006;354:4-7.

Greenhalgh T. How to read a paper: Getting your bearings (deciding what the paper is about). *BMJ.* 1997;315:243-246.

Prentice RL. Measurement error and results from analytic epidemiology: Dietary fat and breast cancer. *J Natl Cancer Inst.* 1996;88:1738-1747.

Spitzer WO, et al. Continuing occurrence of eosinophilia myalgia syndrome in Canada. *Br J Rheumatol.* 1995;34:246-251.

Dietary Fat and Breast Cancer

Boyd NF, et al. A meta-analysis of studies of dietary fat and breast cancer risk. Br J Cancer. 1993;68:627-636.

Greenwald P, Sherwood K, McDonald SS. Fat, caloric intake, and obesity: Lifestyle risk factors for breast cancer. *J Am Diet Assoc.* 1997;97(Suppl):S24-30.

Holmes MD, et al. Association of dietary intake of fat and fatty acids with risk of breast cancer. *JAMA.* 1999;281:914-920.

Prentice RL, et al. Low-fat dietary pattern and risk of invasive breast cancer: the Women's Health Initiative Randomized Controlled Dietary Modification Trial. *JAMA.* 2006;295:629-642.

Thomson CA, et al. Cancer incidence and mortality during the intervention and postintervention periods of the Women's Health Initiative dietary modification trial. *Cancer Epidemiol Biomarkers Prev.* 2014;23:2924-2935.

Martin LJ, et al. A randomized trial of dietary intervention for breast cancer prevention. *Cancer Res.* 2011;71:123-133.

Hunter DJ, et al. Cohort studies of fat intake and the risk of breast cancer—a pooled analysis. *N Engl J Med.*1996;334:356-361.

Wu AH, Pike MC, Stram DO. Meta-analysis: Dietary fat intake, estrogen levels, and the risk of breast cancer. *J Natl Cancer Inst.* 1999;91:529-534.

Cao Y, Hou L, Wang W. Dietary total fat and fatty acids intake, serum fatty acids and risk of breast cancer: A meta-analysis of prospective cohort studies. *Int J Cancer.* 2016;138:1894-1904.

Hooper L , et al. Reduced or modified dietary fat for preventing cardiovascular disease. *Cochrane Database Syst Rev.* 2012:CD002137.

Evidence-based Medicine and Systematic Review

HEALTH SCENARIO

Dr. Block was just told by his nurse that Mr. Green had been "squeezed" into his schedule at lunchtime tomorrow. This appointment is Mr. Green's fifth visit in 9 weeks. Mr. Green is a 54-year-old high school football coach who is being treated for major depression. His wife called, very upset, to make the appointment and told the nurse that "his medicine is just not working, and he is really bad." Mr. Green has tried two different types of antidepressant drugs before his currently prescribed medication. One was changed after 14 days because of its intolerable side effects, and the second was changed after 3 weeks because of a combination of its side effects and a lack of improvement. Dr. Block reviewed Mr. Green's record and pondered what to do next. During a previous discussion about potential treatment options, Mr. Green said that he does not believe in counseling because "he tried it when he lived in Michigan, and it does not work."

Dr. Block must consider the advantages and disadvantages of the available treatment options for this patient: (1) switch to another antidepressant, (2) augment the current antidepressant with a second agent, (3) try to persuade the patient to get counseling in addition to his medication, (4) consider electroconvulsive therapy (ECT), or (5) refer him for repeated transcranial magnetic stimulation (r-TMS) treatment. What to do? Then, he remembers having seen some recent reports on advances in the treatment of depression, and he decides to search for evidence on the comparative effectiveness (CE) of the approaches that he is considering for Mr. Green.

To find a summary of the evidence, he first searches the website of the Agency for Healthcare Research and Quality (AHRQ). He finds a list of Clinician Research Summaries, including one on "Non-pharmacologic Interventions for Treatment-Resistant Depression in Adults" (AHRQ Clinician Research Summaries, 2012). "Great," he thinks, "my problem is solved." Then, he sees that the summary identifies a number of important knowledge gaps in the reviewed studies: (1) information on quality of life is substantially missing from the studies; (2) few of the studies compare non-pharmacologic interventions with each other or with pharmacologic interventions or combinations of treatments; (3) there is almost no evidence on how the CE might differ for patient subgroups that are defined by age or sex; and (4) the studies use inconsistent measures of treatment resistance, clinical outcomes, and adverse events and have short follow-up periods.

When he retrieves the full research report (www. effectivehealthcare.ahrq.gov/trd. cfm), he finds that most of the studies were published before 2008; thus, they are 6 or more years old and not clearly relevant to his current patient. Shaking his head at the clear lack of external validity and relevance of these studies to his clinical problem, he gives up and decides that he will have to spend some time doing more detailed searches for evidence tonight after dinner.

This physician is a problem solver who is approaching the practice of medicine from the perspective of patient-centered care. He knows that different treatments may work differently in different patients and that the most efficacious treatment for a cohort of patients in a clinical trial may not be the most effective or acceptable therapy for a specific patient. He needs quick information on the CE of the therapies that he thinks will be acceptable to his patient. What he needs to do is related to the scope of evidence-based medicine.

EVIDENCE-BASED MEDICINE

Evidence-based medicine (EBM) aims to optimize decision-making by emphasizing the use of the best evidence from well-designed and well-conducted research. In 1996, Professor David Sackett, a Canadian clinical epidemiologist and a pioneer of evidence-based medicine, defined EBM as follows: "Evidence-based medicine is the conscientious, explicit, and judicious use of current best evidence, integrated perfectly with individual clinical expertise and years of clinical experience, and thoughtful identification and compassionate use of individual patients' predicaments, rights, and preferences in making decisions about the care of individual patients." (Sackett et al., 1996) This definition has multiple implications. First, it acknowledges that medical practice in the past was also based on evidence but not necessarily the best evidence referred to in EBM. Second, clinical experience is also regarded as evidence, although it is not systematically collected and is not obtained from well-designed scientific research. Third, the previous practice of medicine was sometimes based on non-scientific evidence, and the approach was often tentative, spontaneous, ambiguous, and not explicit. EBM emphasizes that evidence-based medical practice should be an organized and planned strategy. Fourth, because the subjects of medical research represent a sample from the underlying patient population, the findings reflect the average patient only. The most appropriate clinical decision process requires careful consideration of the specific conditions of each individual patient, taking into account research evidence, the full range of the patient's medical conditions, and the practitioner's clinical experience. When high-quality research evidence is insufficient, personal experience by fault may be the basis for decision-making.

EBM emphasizes a systematic search, evaluation, and application of evidence obtained from scientific investigations as the basis for clinical decisions. When making medical decisions, the current best evidence should be used honestly, conscientiously, explicitly, unambiguously, judiciously, and decisively. The practice of evidence-based medicine involves integrating one's individual clinical expertise with the best available external clinical evidence from systematic research. The foundation of EBM is evidence that is collected from published research articles; these articles are characterized by scientifically rigorous designs, such as **randomized controlled trials (RCTs)**, and are incorporated into systematic reviews and meta-analyses.

Comparative effectiveness research (CER) is a form of EBM (Tanenbaum, 2009). However, while EBM emphasizes that the best evidence comes from well-designed clinical research, such as RCTs, CER chooses the effectiveness of treatments.

The Congressional Budget Office (CBO, 2007) defined CER as follows: **"a rigorous evaluation of the impact of different options that are available for treating a given medical condition for a particular set of patients"** (CBO, 2007 p. 3). A report from the Institute of Medicine (IOM, 2009) that lists the CER topics that should be top priorities for funding also identifies the following four types of research designs that are relevant to CER: (1) systematic reviews and meta-analyses, (2) decision analysis models, (3) **observational studies (OSs)**, and (4) large **pragmatic clinical trials**.

Performing a systematic review, using a decision analysis model, or analyzing observational data from his own patients or from a large health system database is clearly not feasible for informing Dr. Block's treatment decisions in the Health Scenario. Furthermore, he knows that these methodological approaches do not provide the level of evidence that would result from a well-designed and well-executed RCT. It would be ideal if he could find the results of a large pragmatic clinical trial that compared his five treatment choices for middle-aged men who have undergone two previous failed pharmaceutical treatments for depression and who have a history indicating that counseling for depression is not effective. However, such a trial does not exist. Indeed, it may be impossible and unethical to do such a trial, as there is substantial evidence available from individual studies to indicate that ECT (Nahas et al., 2013) and r-TMS (Carpenter et al., 2012) are effective in the majority of patients with treatment-resistant depression and that the augmentation of antidepressants with additional drugs has only a moderate effect in patients with a history of previous drug failures (Fava et al., 2006). Thus, because Dr. Block will have to rely on the reports of effectiveness of treatments that do not use the strongest possible research design to ensure the internal validity of their findings and thus may be affected by selection bias, he needs to know how to judge the quality of the studies that report results using systematic reviews or meta-analyses, decision analysis models, or observational data analyses.

The objectives of this chapter are to introduce the methods used in CER, illustrate when each specific method is used, introduce how to conduct a review and a meta-analysis, and briefly discuss how to (1) avoid selection bias when using observational data to compare effectiveness and (2) integrate the evidence to estimate outcomes that patients care about or outcomes that are expected beyond the observation period using decision analysis modeling.

THE FOUR COMPARATIVE EFFECTIVENESS APPROACHES

The objective of all CER studies is to generate evidence that will help inform day-to-day clinical and health policy decisions. For this reason, CER studies must rely on head-to-head comparisons of active treatments that are used in current practice. These treatments must be used in a study population that is typical of patients with the condition of interest, and the measured outcomes must include those that patients care the most about. This forges a strong link between CER and the research trend toward measuring patient-related outcomes (PROs), and it also focuses on issues like cost and quality, which

are of clear interest to health policymakers. It also ties in recent work on the importance of community engagement for successful research endeavors. The highest quality of evidence will clearly come from CE studies that are designed as large pragmatic clinical trials (LPCTs). However, this design is the costliest to use; it is also the one that takes the longest time to produce new evidence.

LPCT studies have to be large because they compare the effectiveness of two or more treatments used in current clinical practice when we do not know which one is best. Thus, the effect size (treatment difference) is likely to be small, requiring a large number of subjects to be enrolled. Furthermore, the studies have to measure the PRO endpoints that are important to patients and policymakers, limiting the use of surrogate (intermediate) markers for poor clinical outcomes, which are often used in efficacy studies to shorten the time required for patient observation in a trial. The most appropriate study design may be a cluster-randomized trial (Campbell and Walters, 2014) in which each practice or hospital is randomized to a different treatment group to prevent cross-contamination between the treatment groups. It is clear that LPCTs are long and costly, so they are likely to be reserved for CE questions that affect a large number of patients and for cases in which knowing the "best" treatments to choose may have a large impact on both population health and the total cost of care.

This brings us to the "next best" method for generating evidence of the CE of treatments. We can extract clinical trial reports for the treatments of interest and examine how the efficacy of the treatments compares for patient subgroups or across trials using systematic reviews and meta-analyses. A **systematic review** *is a critical assessment and evaluation of all* research studies that address a particular issue. Systematic reviews are carefully structured approaches to extract and examine all the available evidence for and against a treatment. The authors of a systematic review are very careful to minimize bias in their retrieved evidence so that their findings describe the body of evidence that exists to date. Classical meta-analysis has been used for many years to identify a mean treatment effect across sets of studies with inconclusive or inconsistent results (Antman et al., 1992). Some of the early work in this area was done to assess the CE of interventions in obstetrics and perinatal care (Chalmers, 1991), which evolved into the large voluntary research group now known as The Cochrane Collaboration (Chalmers and Hayes, 1994).

There are two problems with meta-analysis: (1) we can only use it to examine treatments with published clinical trial results, and (2) most of the data available will be efficacy data and not data on effectiveness because most clinical trials use stringent inclusion and exclusion criteria for patients and perform treatments in ideal settings, reducing the ability to extrapolate or generalize the results to other patients. Thus, meta-analysis is unlikely to have outcomes that reflect PROs, nor will they be able to examine effectiveness in "real" practice settings. They can also suffer from publication bias because studies with negative findings may be less likely to be published than those with positive findings. However, meta-analysis is very important for its role in examining efficacy in population subgroups and for providing data for the second CER design type: decision analysis modeling.

Decision analysis model is becoming a very important part of CER because it was originally designed to integrate the evidence with the available population and treatment cost data to estimate PROs and the cost of competing treatments under routine practice conditions (Simpson, 1995). Decision analysis is a highly evolved, specialized discipline that has been used for years to compare the health and economic implications of competing therapies. It has proven especially useful for assessing new drugs and for predicting the long-term outcomes of public health interventions, such as screening programs or vaccine use. Very large and complex validated decision analysis models have been constructed to estimate the long-term expected outcomes of diabetes treatments (The Mount Hood Modeling Group, 2007), cancer screening (Eddy et al., 1988), antiretroviral therapy in HIV-disease (Simpson, 2010), vaccine use (Clark et al., 2013), and many other types of interventions. Different structural frameworks and time horizons may be used to organize the available evidence and to test the assumptions embedded in a decision model. The options range from simple decision trees to complex statistical models, and they may use combinations of structures as well as probabilistic approaches, such as simulation modeling, to examine the effects of uncertainty in the evidence on the study outcome.

A well-executed complex decision model may take a large team of clinical, statistical, epidemiologic, economic, and computer science experts several years to build and validate. Many practical (but fairly simple) CE models capture the mean efficacy measures identified in a meta-analysis, adjust them to the expected effectiveness, and link the surrogate outcomes from clinical trials to epidemiologic and health care resource use with data from OSs in relevant patient subgroups. Two separate issues can affect the validity of these CE models: (1) Is the model structure valid? and (2) Are the observational data used to estimate the model drivers affected by selection bias? The issue of **selection bias** is crucial for the validity of decision analysis modeling or for any CE analysis that uses observational data.

Observational studies use data that are generated from treating patients in routine practice settings. This means that the data have excellent generalizability: they clearly represent the patients who one may expect to see in real practice. When these data are used to compare the effectiveness of competing therapies, however, they are very vulnerable to confounding by indication or selection bias. This bias is injected by the fact that practicing physicians will tend to use the newest or best treatment available for their more severely ill or difficult-to-treat patients. Thus, if one simply compares the outcomes for patients treated with treatment A with those treated with treatment B, it is very likely that one group of patients will have more severe disease, be more difficult to treat, or have many more comorbid conditions that affect their treatment outcome. Thus, one would be comparing "apples to oranges." Indeed, this is the reason that patients are randomized in clinical trials. Only if we assign patients to a treatment by chance can we be assured that disease severity, treatment difficulty, comorbidities, demographic characteristics, and any unknown prognostic factors are equally distributed in the treatment groups. However, many important questions in medical care cannot be examined in randomized studies. In some situations, randomized studies may be too expensive to undertake, impractical or infeasible, unethical to perform, or some combination of all of these factors. For these situations, the use of prospectively or retrospectively collected observational data offers an alternative. In such situations, it is essential to use study designs that help guard against selection bias. Two "pseudo-randomization" study design approaches have been developed and validated over the past 20 years using either propensity score (PS) methods or instrumental variable design. Although no OS can completely assure the absence of selection bias, the newest methods, when combined with a sensitivity analysis, do a very good job of removing most of the bias and showing how large the "missed" biasing factor would have to be to nullify the results.

SYSTEMATIC REVIEWS: UTILITY AND DEFINITION

There are many definitions of a systematic review (SR) in the literature and in use by various professional, research, and guideline development groups. We use the following definition, which was adapted from one proposed by the Agency for Healthcare Research and Quality (AHRQ): an SR is a critical assessment and evaluation of all research studies that address a particular issue (http://effectivehealthcare.ahrq.gov/glossary-of-terms/? pageaction=showterm&termid=70) (AHRQ, n.d.b.).

Researchers and other persons developing an SR (review developers) use an organized method of locating, assembling, and evaluating a body of literature on a particular topic using a set of specific criteria. A SR typically includes a description of the findings of the collection of research studies, and it may tailor its presentation of the findings for specific target audiences, including the general public (http://effectivehealthcare.ahrq.gov/glossary-of-terms/?pageaction=showterm&termid=70) (AHRQ, n.d.b.).

Research studies that have been published in peer-reviewed sources are usually the foundational literature for an SR, but other types of literature may also be included, such as "grey" or unpublished literature. Grey literature may include unpublished manuscripts, manuscripts in press, clinical trial registries, conference papers, conference posters, evaluation reports, and grant close-out reports. Searches may be conducted by reviewing grey literature databases (i.e., the Grey Literature Report by The New York Academy of Medicine at http://www.greylit.org, Trip at http://www.tripdatabase.com, DocuTicker at http://www.docuticker.com, or U.S. Government Documents at http://guides.library.upenn.edu/usgovdocuments) or by contacting the authors of published work on the topic or others known to have a special interest in the topic. SR developers include grey literature to help balance the publication bias for a review, as reviews are often biased in favor of randomized controlled trials or positive research findings.

The literature found in an SR may be analyzed in different ways, depending on the outcome of interest, the type of studies included in the review, and the presentation of results. Options range from a narrative qualitative summary of review findings to quantitative pooling of data using meta-analytic statistical techniques.

In summary, SRs are an important tool for health care decision makers and other stakeholders in the health care system. These reviews offer the best summary of existing evidence about a specific topic or set of interventions based on the available literature. SRs identify, select, assess, and synthesize the findings of similar but separate studies and can help clarify what is known and not known about the potential benefits and harms of drugs, devices, and other health care services as well as behavioral and policy-based approaches to improving health and health care. SRs can be helpful for clinicians who want to integrate research findings into their daily practices, for patients who want to make well-informed choices about their own care, and for professional medical societies who are preparing guidance for their members, funders, and policymakers (Institute of Medicine [IOM], 2011).

SYSTEMATIC REVIEWS: PLANNING AN SR

Many organizations offer guidance on how to create a plan for the conduct of an SR. We present an adaptation of several of these approaches by starting with a statement of the intended outcomes of the planning process itself and the use of existing reviews in deciding whether to plan and conduct a review.

OUTCOMES OF A PLANNING PROCESS FOR A SYSTEMATIC REVIEW

The review planning process should result in at least the following three outcomes:

1. *A well-framed question or set of questions* specifying the types of populations or participants, interventions, comparisons, and outcomes (PICO) to be included in the review. The specification of these types of information to frame the review is often referred to as the PICO for the SR (Higgins and Green, 2011; IOM, 2011).

2. *A statement on what types of studies* are to be included in the review (e.g., clinical trials and observational studies, among others).

3. A description (often a logic model or analytic framework) that describes the relationship of the PICO elements with one another.

Decisions about these outcomes of the planning process frame the review and become the pre-specified eligibility criteria for including specific studies in the review.

SEARCH FOR EXISTING REVIEWS

Many organizations conduct SRs on a wide range of health and health care topics (**Table 11-1**). Anyone considering the conduct of a review would be well advised to search these and other available sources to determine whether a timely SR has been done on the topic or question of interest. An existing review would be most helpful if it was found to:

- Answer the same key question(s) of interest
- Provide appropriate and timely information
- Offer feasible and reasonable approaches to answering the key question(s), solving a simi-

Table 11-1 Selected organizations producing systematic reviews.

SR Developers	Website
International:	
The Cochrane Collaboration	http://www.cochrane.org/
Centre for Reviews & Dissemination (CRD)	http://www.york.ac.uk/inst/crd/
The Campbell Collaboration	http://www.campbellcollaboration.org/
National Institute for Health & Clinical Excellence (NICE)	http://www.nice.org.uk/
US Private:	
BCBS Association Technology Evaluation Center	http://www.ahrq.gov/research/findings/ evidence-based-reports/centers/bcbsatec.html
ECRI Institute	https://www.ecri.org/Pages/default.aspx
Hayes International, Inc.	http://www.haynesintl.com/
U.S. Government:	
AHRQ Effective Health Care Program via Evidence-based Practice Centers	http://www.ahrq.gov/research/findings/ evidence-based-reports/overview/index.html
Centers for Disease Control and Prevention (CDC)	http://www.cdc.gov/
The Substance Abuse and Mental Health Services Administration (SAMHSA)	http://www.samhsa.gov/

Data from Institute of Medicine. (2011). *Finding What Works in Health Care: Standards for Systematic Reviews.* Washington, DC: The National Academies

lar problem, or meeting specific needs

- Represent findings from similar situations or settings or among similar populations
- Use best practices to conduct the review and report its findings
- Engage relevant stakeholders in the design, conduct, and interpretation of the review findings

If the search identifies a review that meets most of these criteria, its findings may be adequate to answer the question at hand, prompt the implementation of findings in a specific setting, "tee up" research based on the research gaps identified in the review, or inform program or policy design.

If the identified reviews do not include recent literature on the key question(s), the review developer may choose to update the existing review. In this case, the review developer may have a significantly shortened planning process because it should be possible (and preferable) to replicate the prior review's SR protocol as closely as possible with at least one notable exception, the inclusion dates for the review. The new review should start where the prior review ended and continue to the most recent, reasonable date. After searches for the new review are complete, the analysis can be replicated either by combining all the data, as would be necessary for a meta-analysis, or by examining the new findings and then doing a cross-walk with the findings of the existing review, an approach that is more suited to a qualitative synthesis strategy for determining review findings.

If the search for reviews is unsuccessful, the review developer may elect to complete a planning process for a new SR, taking into account the resources that are necessary to conduct the review and the research developer's capacity to undertake the review. Reviews of complex questions can be quite expensive and time consuming, so a consideration of the costs and time constraints is very important in deciding to conduct a review. Each of these steps requires a consideration of how financial support will be obtained to cover the time that individuals spend on the SR and the other expenses that are associated with the review, such as article retrieval.

PLAN DEVELOPMENT STEPS

The methods and processes to create an SR plan are recommended by the primary developers of SRs. We present our adaptation of the IOM Standards for Systematic Reviews (2011) as an orientation to the essential components of an SR plan. It is vitally important to document the decisions that are made in each step so that the chosen approaches can be described in the presentation of the SR findings. More details on how to approach each step can be found at www.nationalacademies.org/hmd/Reports/2011/Finding-What-Works-in-Health-Care-Standards-for-Systematic-Reviews/Standards.aspx (IOM, 2011).

We offer approaches to each of the seven steps that are necessary to plan a "new" review.

Step 1

The first step is to establish a team with the appropriate expertise and experience to conduct the SR. The team should include individuals with expertise in the pertinent content areas; SR methods, searching for relevant evidence, quantitative and qualitative methods; and other expertise, as appropriate.

Approach: The researcher may identify members of an SR team with experience in designing and conducting an SR and in the methods necessary to conduct an SR. Individuals may be invited to join the team based on their experience in relevant content areas. A research librarian with experience in conducting searches for an SR or on complex topics would be recruited along with a researcher who is well-versed in the use of qualitative methods. This SR is unlikely to need an expert in quantitative methods, such as meta-analysis, given the type of literature on this topic.

Step 2

The second step is to manage the bias and conflict of interest (COI) of the SR team conducting the SR. A process should be established to require each team member to disclose their potential COI and professional or intellectual bias, exclude individuals with a clear financial conflict, and exclude individuals whose professional or intellectual bias would diminish the credibility of the review in the eyes of the intended users.

Approach: Most academic institutions have COI processes in place, and if all team members are part of that process, the team leader may proceed to document any reported COI or inquire about any further COI that may be present given the location, content area, or scope of the SR. For any members of the team whose organizations do not require a COI, the team leader should establish a process for identifying and documenting the COI. In some cases, it may be necessary to reconsider the membership of a specific team member based on his or her declared COI.

Step 3

The third step is to ensure user and stakeholder input as the review is designed and conducted. Although user and stakeholder input is vital to planning the review, a process should be in place to protect the independence of the review team in making the final decisions about the design, analysis, and reporting of the review.

Recent efforts by the Patient Centered Outcomes Research Institute (PCORI) and others seek to assure greater transparency of the SR processes and to engage patients and other stakeholders in the review process. Stakeholder groups are variously identified by SR developers, but they are generally assumed, in the areas of health and health care, to include patients and their caregivers; clinicians, including physicians, nurses, and other health care professionals; payers; and policymakers, including guideline developers and other SR sponsors.

Patient and stakeholder involvement in each step of the SR process is critical. Their perspectives inform the development of key questions, primary and secondary outcomes, analytic frameworks, strength of evidence, and interpretation of findings. Including these perspectives helps to ensure that the reviews address outcomes that are meaningful to

patients and other stakeholders and provide actionable recommendations for all stakeholder groups and their members.

Stakeholder participation may be hampered by their awareness and understanding of the methods used to conduct an SR; their bias for or against SR processes, findings, and applications; their interpretation of the implications of the review findings for themselves and their organizations; and their understanding of their role in the SR process.

The principles of community engagement can be applied to increase the quality of stakeholder involvement in SR processes. Stakeholders can be offered orientation sessions describing their roles and responsibilities as stakeholder advisory panel members. They can also be offered training to increase their knowledge of the SR process and appreciate the strengths and limitations of an SR. Materials associated with planning the SR can be presented in "plain language," and ample time can be given for discussion or clarification.

Just as stakeholders may need to gain familiarity with the SR process, some review team members may need to learn more about the contextual factors and other factors affecting the topic of the review from the stakeholder perspective. This bidirectional learning is likely to enhance the relevance, credibility, and acceptance of review findings.

Step 4

The fourth step is to manage the bias and COI of the individuals who are providing input into the SR. Similar to the process for the COI of review team members, individuals providing input on the review should be required, through a transparent, consistently used and applied process, to disclose any potential COI and professional or intellectual bias. The process should include an approach to identifying and excluding individuals whose COI or bias would diminish the credibility of the SR in the eyes of the intended users.

Approach: The review team's point of contact will develop, with stakeholder input, a process for assuring the identification and disclosure of any COI for the members of the stakeholder advisory panel.

Step 5

Formulate the topic of the SR. In this step, the review team should confirm the need for a new review and develop an analytic framework that clearly lays out the chain of logic linking the health intervention to the outcomes of interest and defining the key questions to be addressed by the SR. A standard format to articulate each question of interest should be developed, and it should state the rationale for each question. Key questions should be shared with the intended users and stakeholders and refined, if necessary, based on their input. The types of questions may encompass clinical, behavioral, systems, or policy concerns in a particular field (IOM, 2011).

Step 6

The sixth step is to develop an SR protocol describing the following elements of the SR process:

1. The context and rationale for the SR, from both a decision-making and a research perspective

2. The study screening and selection criteria (inclusion and exclusion criteria)

3. The precise outcome measures, time points, interventions, and comparison groups to be addressed

4. The search strategy for identifying relevant evidence

5. The procedures for study selection

6. The data extraction strategy

7. The process for identifying and resolving disagreements between the researchers in study selection and data extraction decisions

8. The approach to critically appraise individual studies

9. The method for evaluating the body of evidence, including the quantitative and qualitative synthesis strategies

10. Any planned analyses of differential treatment effects according to patient subgroups, how an intervention is delivered, or how an outcome is measured

11. The proposed timetable for conducting the review

12. The conduct and timing of a public comment period for the protocol and a public report on the disposition of comments (IOM, 2011)

Approach: The review team develops a draft of the protocol in consultation with its expert members and with input from the stakeholder advisory panel, as necessary.

Step 7

The seventh step is to submit the protocol for peer review.

QUANTITATIVE SYSTEMATIC REVIEW DEFINITION

The **systematic review** plays a central role in modern health care delivery. In particular, quantitative systematic reviews (also known as meta-analyses), which combine multiple studies with similar characteristics to achieve vastly greater statistical power and precision than can be obtained in any one study, can settle controversies from conflicting studies and inform clinical guidelines and health care decisions.

Methods to conduct systematic reviews include both quantitative and qualitative approaches. Both approaches offer advantages and disadvantages, and their use often is predicated upon the types of studies available to answer a specific question.

PERFORMING A QUANTITATIVE SYSTEMATIC REVIEW: META-ANALYSIS

When the study designs, populations, treatments or interventions, exposures, and outcomes (including how and when these were assessed) of the studies included in the systematic review are similar, it is possible to summarize the published evidence quantitatively (using statistical methods) by performing a meta-analysis. The key components of a meta-analysis are as follows:

- A clearly stated set of objectives with predefined eligibility criteria for the studies
- An explicit, reproducible methodology

- A systematic search that attempts to capture all studies that would meet the eligibility criteria
- An assessment of the validity of the findings of the included studies (e.g., through an assessment of the risk of bias)
- A systematic presentation and synthesis of the characteristics and findings of the included studies

A meta-analysis should be executed, step-by-step, using the following framework and steps:

1. Search strategy: The search strategy should be based on the main concepts being examined. The terms to be used to conduct the literature search should be determined by the study hypothesis, the research questions, and the database in which the search is to be conducted. Moreover, the search should be reproducible. An experienced medical librarian can be invaluable in designing and executing a comprehensive search. The specification of search terms should be vetted thoroughly with the review team to ensure that the appropriate studies are identified and that a systematic bias related to the search criteria is avoided. Please see Chapter 10 for detailed information on how to build a search strategy in PubMed.

2. Inclusion/exclusion (I/E) criteria: A key feature of a systematic review is the pre-specification of criteria for including and excluding studies in the review (eligibility criteria). For the search strategy, the I/E criteria should be based on the study hypothesis and research questions. Features of the target population to whom the results of the systematic review are intended to apply should also be considered in determining the study I/E criteria so that the findings can be generalized (external validity) accordingly. For example, if the systematic review is intended to inform the development of clinical guidelines for the treatment of coronary artery disease in elderly adults, a study in which enrollment was limited to patients under 50 years of age should not be included, as its results are not relevant to the systematic review's purpose. The I/E criteria also impact the systematic review's internal valid-

ity; for example, including non-RCT studies that do not rigorously account for confounding factors or excluding RCT studies that have a high crossover rate (even if the analysis was correctly executed using an *intention-to-treat* approach) might significantly bias the meta-analysis findings.

Inclusion of non-RCT studies in a meta-analysis: By definition, a meta-analysis is a summary of all the empirical evidence that is associated with the specific research question. Therefore, it is critical to consider all rigorous and well-executed studies, including non-RCTs, on the topic of interest. Rigorously adjusted (by recognized confounders and other possible confounders of the association of interest) non-RCTs provide critical evidence on the impact of the intervention or exposure on the evaluated outcome in a real-world setting. Although RCTs continue to be considered the gold standard in empirical research, they suffer from one very important weakness, limited external validity (generalizability) because of their narrow inclusion criteria; this creates a difficulty in translating the study findings beyond the evaluated experimental cohort. The inclusion of non-RCTs in the meta-analysis helps address this lack of external validity. Accordingly, both RCTs and non-RCTs should be considered in a meta-analysis, and the findings should be presented by study type and overall.

3. Data abstraction: The processes used to abstract the data from the articles considered in the meta-analysis are critical and should be designed to warrant the highest validity and reliability of the collected information. A standardized data collection tool that clearly specifies exactly what information needs to be collected from each article should be created and used by the research team that is abstracting the data.

4. Assessment of risk of bias: The internal validity of the meta-analysis depends on whether the data and results from the included studies are valid (i.e., the studies were conducted rigorously) and generalizable. Accordingly, a meta-analysis of the poor-quality studies will have low internal validity and is likely to produce biased results. The evaluation of the risk of bias of the included studies is critical because it influences the interpretation of the studies and the conclusions of the review.

The specifics on how to collect and report the risk of bias in the data depend very much on the tool chosen to assess it. A good option, particularly when all or most of the included studies are RCTs, is the Cochrane Collaboration's RCT Bias Assessment Tool (see http://handbook.cochrane.org/chapter_8/table_8_5_a_the_cochrane_collaborations_tool_for_assessing.htm), in which the risk of bias in a specified set of categories is judged to be at low, high, or unclear risk. Other tools may be more appropriate when focusing on observational studies, and when both RCTs and observational studies are included in the same systematic review, some adaptation may be required to enable one tool to be consistently applied across all the studies.

5. Publication bias: In some instances, a study's publication is affected by its findings; most commonly, this takes the form of studies that show non-significant associations between the intervention and the outcome of interest, which results in the work not reaching publication. Publication bias is an important issue to consider when conducting a systematic review because the internal validity of the systematic review heavily depends on the evidence included in (or omitted from) the review. Because the researcher conducting a systematic review seldom has any practical means of determining which studies have remained unpublished, let alone any means of obtaining their results, the reporting bias frequently has to be assessed solely based on the published studies. This can be done via a scatter plot (funnel plot) that depicts the intervention effect estimates from the individual studies against some measure of each study's size or precision. An asymmetrical plot suggests that a publication bias may be present (i.e., some studies showing non-statistically significant effects are not published).

6. Measures of association (statistical analysis and data synthesis): Estimation of the measures of association depends on the type of outcome: binary, continuous, categorical (more than two level out-

come) or ordinal, counts or rates, or time to event. **Table 11-2** summarizes the measures of association for each type of outcome.

Table 11-2 Systematic review measures of association by outcome

Type of Outcome	Measure of Association
Binary	Risk ratio
	Odds ratio
	Risk difference
Continuous	Mean difference
	Standardized mean difference
Ordinal	Proportional odds ratio
Counts or rate	Rate ratio
Time to event	Hazard ratio

7. Heterogeneity: The intervention effects of the studies included in a meta-analysis might vary because of random error alone or due to differences in the studies' methodologies (e.g., outcome assessment procedures, study population, study design). This variation is commonly known as heterogeneity. When the intervention effects show **different directions** and magnitudes between the studies, the heterogeneity is more likely to be attributable to methodological differences between the studies, and a meta-analysis **cannot** be performed. In this case, a qualitative review of the evidence may be presented instead. By contrast, when the intervention effects have the **same direction** but different magnitudes between the studies, the heterogeneity is more likely to be attributable to chance, and it is appropriate to conduct a meta-analysis to summarize the available evidence.

8. Sensitivity analysis: Performing a meta-analysis involves a series of decisions, specifically, choosing a search strategy, the study I/E criteria, and the measures of association that are of interest; assessing the sources of heterogeneity (and deciding whether a meta-analysis is appropriate); and choosing the types of sensitivity analysis that need to be performed. In some situations, these decisions might be arbitrary, making the meta-analysis findings susceptible to bias. To assess whether the meta-analysis results are independent from the investigator's decisions, a sensitivity analysis should be performed by repeating the primary analysis and substituting alternative decisions that were arbitrary or unclear (e.g., include the excluded studies in the analysis).

9. Presentation of results: A very intuitive and clear way of presenting findings from a meta-analysis is with a Forest plot. The Forest plot shows the overall effect (and associated 95% CI) that is estimated from the meta-analysis as well as the raw summary data for each included study, including the total number of patients by intervention or control group, the total number of events (mean and standard deviation are used for continuous outcomes) by intervention or control group, the percent weight (the "weight" the individual study contributes to the overall effect), and the weighted (depending on the cohort size) point estimate (i.e., intervention effect). Revman 5.2 further automatically includes the results of a heterogeneity test, a chi-squared statistic, and a test for differences across subgroups in the Forest plot, which aid in interpretation.

Finally, when writing up the systematic review for publication, the standards laid out in the Preferred Reporting Items for Systematic Reviews and Meta-Analysis (PRISMA) Statement should be followed. Most peer-reviewed journal articles require this standard (including submission of the PRISMA checklist) for publication. Details on the PRISMA statement, including the PRISMA checklist and a template for creating the flow diagram of the studies that are included and excluded in the systematic review, are available at http://www.prismastatement.org.

It is a good idea to consult the PRISMA checklist at the start of the systematic review process to ensure that one records all of the information necessary to comply with the PRISMA standards (e.g., reasons why studies were excluded) along the way.

SUMMARY

As a form of evidence-based medicine (EBM), **comparative effectiveness research (CER)** has been defined as a "rigorous evaluation of the impact of

different options that are available for treating a given medical condition" (CBO, 2007). The following four types of research designs fall within the domain of CER: (1) systematic review or quantitative synthesis, (2) decision analysis, (3) OSs, and (4) large pragmatic clinical trials. In this chapter, we have explored how these various designs can contribute to informing treatment selection.

Large pragmatic clinical trials offer the advantage of providing the highest quality of evidence because they randomize patients across the treatment alternatives that are under consideration. Unfortunately, large RCTs are expensive to conduct, take comparatively long to complete, and often have restrictive inclusion criteria, making it difficult to extrapolate their findings to other patient populations.

In this chapter, we have illustrated how to conduct an SR or a meta-analysis. An SR is a critical assessment and evaluation of all the research studies that address a particular issue. Typically, an SR relies principally on the results of investigations that are published in the peer-reviewed literature, but they may also include "grey" literature (e.g., unpublished manuscripts, conference papers and posters, grant close-out reports). The findings of an SR may be summarized in a variety of ways, ranging from a qualitative assessment to a formal statistical summary, referred to as a meta-analysis. The planning and execution of a formal SR should follow well-established guidelines, including focusing on the topic of interest, assembling an inter-professional team to work together, identifying potential stakeholders from various interested parties and soliciting their input, identifying and managing any conflicts of interest, developing a protocol, and submitting the protocol for peer review. In the following chapters, the elements of performing an SR are presented in detail. A meta-analysis or quantitative synthesis generally provides high-quality information, particularly when summarizing RCT data, but it is often limited to the published literature, which may be biased toward studies with positive results. The ability to extrapolate data to populations that are similar to those encountered in "real–world" clinical practice also may be limited.

Models based on decision analysis are becoming more widely used because they can incorporate large and complex data that reflect routine clinical care situations. A variety of methods can be used for decision analysis purposes, ranging from relatively simple decision trees to complex models. Fundamental to interpreting the results of a decision analysis is affirming both that (1) the structure of the model is valid and that (2) the data used in the model are free from bias or other errors.

Observational data may be limited by potential sources of bias that are related to the absence of randomization of the treatment assignment. However, data from these studies may represent the typical clinical practice setting more appropriately than the constrained parameters of a clinical trial. Observational data are also available on a wide range of topics from routinely collected data and therefore may be much less expensive and time consuming for the investigator to amass.

Observational data sources include clinical record systems as well as the administrative data used for billing and regulatory purposes. These data sources often include very large patient populations that are followed over time. The lack of randomization, however, raises the question of whether the compared treatment groups are balanced with respect to both known and unknown prognostic factors. A variety of methods have been developed to "pseudo-randomize" the study subjects, that is, to mathematically eliminate any potential bias in the underlying differences between the compared groups.

Comparative effectiveness research is becoming an increasingly important approach for the evaluation of treatment options and decision-making on optimal care. The ability to interpret the results of CER will emerge as a crucial skill for clinicians, regardless of the care setting and focus of practice.

(Tao Wu)

IMPORTANT TERMINOLOGY

evidence-based medicine (EBM)　循证医学

randomized controlled trials (RCTs)　随机对照试验

comparative effectiveness research　疗效对比研究

observational studies (OSs)　观察性研究

pragmatic clinical trials　实用性临床试验

systematic review　系统综述

decision analysis model　决策分析模型

selection bias　选择偏倚

 STUDY QUESTIONS

1. What is one of the weaknesses related to meta-analyses?

A. *They combine information from multiple studies.*

B. *Most of the data available will be efficacy data, not data on effectiveness.*

C. *Similar endpoints from multiple studies are used to generate a combined effect size.*

D. *They are not well accepted.*

2. Which of these is NOT a strength of observational studies?

A. *Their longitudinal nature or ability for researchers to follow patients over very long periods of time, which are most often contiguous.*

B. *Their ready availability at little expense.*

C. *Their ability to control for selection bias with the randomization of subjects.*

D. *Their ability to answer research questions that cannot be answered with RCTs, such as the effects of changes in policy or clinical practice.*

3. A systematic review is

A. *a critical assessment and evaluation of all the research studies that address a particular issue.*

B. *a review of the literature on a topic that is relevant to health and health care.*

C. *always a meta-analysis.*

D. *a fair and balanced way to review available evidence.*

4. PICO stands for

A. *patients, interventions, consultations, and outcomes.*

B. *populations, inventions, comparisons, and observation.*

C. populations, interventions, comparisons, and outcomes.

D. patients, inventions, comorbidities, and outcomes.

5. What should be considered when determining the
search strategy for a meta-analysis?

A. The time that it will take to read the manuscripts
identified from the search.

B. The study hypothesis and the number of possible
studies that the search will return.

C. The study hypothesis, research questions, and the
database in which the search is to be conducted.

D. The research questions and the number of possible
studies that the search will return.

FURTHER READING

Evidence-Based Medicine and Comparative Effectiveness:

Austin PC. The relative ability of different propensity score
methods to balance measured covariates between treated
and untreated subjects in observational studies. *Med Decis
Making.* 2009;29(6):661-677.

Evidence-Based Medicine Working Group. Evidence-based
medicine. A new approach to teaching the practice of
medicine. *JAMA.* 1992;268(17):2420-2425.

Meyer AM, Wheeler SB, Weinberger M, et al. An overview of
methods for comparative effectiveness research. *Semin
Radiat Oncol.* 2014;24: 5-13.

Mitchell JB, Bubolz T, Paul JE, et al. Using Medicare claims for
outcomes research. *Med Care.* 1994;32(7 suppl):JS38-JS51.

Sher DJ, Punglia RS. Decision analysis and cost effectiveness
research—a primer. *Semin Radiat Oncol.* 2014;24: 14-24.

Systematic Review and Meta-Analysis:

Higgins JPT, Green S. Cochrane Handbook for Systematic
Reviews of Interventions Version 5.1.0 [updated March
2011]. The Cochrane Collaboration. Published 2011.
http://www.cochrane-handbook.org.

Ioannidis JP, Patsopoulos, Evangelou E. Uncertainty in heterogeneity estimates in meta-analyses. *BMJ.* 2007;335:
914-916.

Moher D, Liberati A, Tetzlaff J, et al.The PRISMA Group.
Preferred reporting items for systematic reviews and

meta-analysis: the PRISMA statement. *Ann Intern Med.*
2009;151(4):264-269.

Moher D, Liberati A, Tetzlaff J, Altman DG; The PRISMA
Group. Preferred reporting items for systematic reviews
and meta-analysis: the PRISMA statement. *PLoS Med.*
2009;6(6): e1000097.

Thompson SG, Higgins JP. How should meta-regression analyses be undertaken and interpreted? *Stat Med.* 2002;21:
1559-1573.

REFERENCES

Evidence-Based Medicine and Comparative Effectiveness:

AHRQ Clinician Research Summaries. (2012, March). Non-
pharmacologic interventions for treatment-resistant
depression in adults. Pub.11(12)-EHC056-3.

Antman EM, Lau J, Kulpenick B, et al. A comparison of results
of meta-analysis of randomized controlled trials and recommendations of clinical experts: treatments for myocardial infarction. *JAMA.* 1992; 268:240-248.

Campbell MJ, Walters SJ. How to Design, Analyze, and Report
Cluster Randomized Trials. Hoboken, NJ: Wiley; 2014.

Carpenter LL, Janicak PG, Aaronson ST, et al. Transcranial
magnetic stimulation (TMS) for major depression: a
multisite, naturalistic, observational study of acute treatment outcomes in clinical practice. *Depress Anxiety.*
2012;29(7):587-596.

Chalmers I, Hayes B. Systematic reviews: reporting, updating,
and correcting systematic reviews of effects of health care.
BMJ. 1994; 309:862.

Chalmers I. The work of the National Perinatal Epidemiology
Unit. One example of technology assessment in perinatal
care. *Int J Technol Assess Health Care.* 1991;7(4):430-459.

Clark A, Jaurequi B, Griffith U, et al. TRIVAC decision-sup-
port model for evaluating the cost-effectiveness of Hae-
mophilus influenza type b, pneumococcal and rotavirus
vaccination. *Vaccine.* 2013;31(suppl 3):C19-C29.

Congressional Budget Office. Research on the comparative
effectiveness of medical treatments. December, 2007.
www.cbo.gov/ publication/41655. Accessed on May 10,
2014.

Eddy DM, Hasselblad V, McGivney W, et al. The value of
mammography screening in women under age 50. *JAMA.*
1988; 259:1512-1519.

Fava M, Rush AJ, Wisniewski SR, et al. A comparison of mirtazapine and nortriptyline following two consecutive failed medication treatments for depressed outpatients: a STAR*D report. *Am J Psychiatry*. 2006;163(7):1161-1172.

Institute of Medicine. Initial national priorities for comparative effectiveness research. Report Brief June, 2009. www.iom.edu/cerpriorities. Accessed on May 10, 2014.

Nahas Z, Short B, Burns C, et al. A feasibility study of a new method for electrically producing seizures in man: focal electrically administered seizure therapy [FEAST]. *Brain Stimul*. 2013;6(3):403-408

Sackett DL, Rosenberg WM, Gray JA, et al. Evidence based medicine: what it is and what it isn't. *BMJ*. 1996;312(7023):71-72.

Simpson KN. Economic modeling of HIV treatments. *Curr Opin HIV AIDS*. 2010;5(3):242-248.

Simpson KN. Modeling with clinical trial data: getting from the data researchers have to the data decision makers need. *Drug Info J*. 1995;29(4):1431-1440.

Tanenbaum SJ. Comparative effectiveness research: evidence-based medicine meets health care reform in the USA. *J Eval Clin Pract*. 2009;15(6):976-984.

The Mount Hood Modeling Group. Computer Modeling of Diabetes and Its Complications: A report on the Fourth Mount Hood Challenge Meeting. *Diabetes care*. 2007;30(6): 1638-1646.

Zhan C, Miller MR. Administrative data based patient safety research: a critical review. *Qual Saf Health Care*. 2003;12(suppl 2): ii58-ii63.

Systematic Review:

Agency for Healthcare Research and Quality. Meta-analysis. In Glossary of Terms. http://effectivehealthcare.ahrq.gov/glossaryof-terms/?pageaction=showterm&termid=39. Published n.d.a. Accessed June 4, 2014.

Agency for Healthcare Research and Quality. Systematic review. In Glossary of Terms. http://effectivehealthcare.ahrq.gov/glossaryof-terms/?pageaction=showterm&termid=70. Published n.d.b. Accessed June 4, 2014.

Higgins JT, Green S, eds. Cochrane Handbook for Systematic Reviews of Interventions Version 5.1.0. Published March, 2011. http://www.cochrane-handbook.org. Accessed June 4, 2014.

Institute of Medicine. (2011). Finding What Works in Health Care: Standards for systematic Reviews. Washington, DC: National Academies Press. South Carolina Department of Health and Environmental Control, Bureau of Community Health and Chronic Disease Prevention. County Chronic Disease Fact Sheet. Published November, 2013. http://www.scdhec.gov/hs/epidata/county_reports.htm. Accessed June 4, 2014.

Definition of a Systematic Review

Cochrane AL. Archie Cochrane in his own words. Selections arranged from his 1972 introduction to "Effectiveness and Efficiency: Random Reflections on the Health Services" 1972. *Control Clin Trials*. 1989;10(4):428-433.

Performing a Quantitative Systematic Review: Meta-Analysis

Harrell FE Jr. Regression Modeling Strategies: With Application to Linear Models, Logistic Regression, and Survival Analysis. New York: Springer-Verlag; 2001.

Higgins JP, Altman DG, Gotzsche PC, et al. The Cochrane Collaboration's tool for assessing risk of bias in randomised trials. *BMJ*. 2011;343: d5928.

Higgins JPT, Green S, eds. Cochrane Handbook for Systematic Reviews of Interventions Version 5.1.0 [updated March 2011]. The Cochrane Collaboration. Published 2011. http://www.cochrane-handbook.org.

Review Manager (RevMan) [Computer program]. Version 5.3. Copenhagen: The Nordic Cochrane Centre, The Cochrane Collaboration; 2012.U.S. National Library of Medicine. PubMed.gov.

Communicable Disease Epidemiology

12

HEALTH SCENARIO

The Ebola virus causes an acute, serious illness which is often fatal if untreated. Ebola virus disease (EVD) first appeared in 1976 in 2 simultaneous outbreaks, one in what is now, Nzara, South Sudan, and the other in Yambuku, Democratic Republic of Congo. The latter occurred in a village near the Ebola River, from which the disease takes its name.

The current outbreak in West Africa, (first cases notified in March 2014), is the largest and most complex Ebola outbreak since the Ebola virus was first discovered in 1976. There have been more cases and deaths in this outbreak than all others combined. It has also spread between countries starting in Guinea then spreading across land borders to Sierra Leone and Liberia, by air to Nigeria and USA, and by land to Senegal and Mali.

The most severely affected countries, Guinea, Liberia and Sierra Leone, have very weak health systems, lack human and infrastructural resources, and have only recently emerged from long periods of conflict and instability. On August 8, the World Health Organization (WHO) Director-General declared the West Africa outbreak a Public Health Emergency of International Concern under the International Health Regulations.

There are five species of Ebola virus that have been identified: Zaire, Bundibugyo, Sudan, Reston and Taï Forest. The first three, Bundibugyo ebola virus, Zaire ebola virus, and Sudan ebola virus have been associated with large outbreaks in Africa. The virus causing the 2014 West African outbreak belongs to the Zaire species.

The virus is transmitted to people from wild animals and spreads in the human population through human-to-human transmission. The average EVD case fatality rate is around 50%. Case fatality rates have varied from 25% to 90% in past outbreaks. The first EVD outbreaks occurred in remote villages in Central Africa, near tropical rainforests, but the most recent outbreak in West Africa has involved major urban as well as rural areas. Community engagement is key to successfully controlling outbreaks. Good outbreak control relies on applying a package of interventions, namely case management, surveillance and contact tracing, a good laboratory service, safe burials and social mobilization. There are currently no licensed Ebola vaccines but 2 potential candidates are undergoing evaluation.

INTRODUCTION

It is often said that epidemiology is the basic science of preventive medicine. To prevent diseases, it is important to understand the causative agents, risk factors and circumstances that lead to a specific disease. This is especially important for communicable disease prevention, since simple interventions may break the chain of transmission.

INFECTIOUS, COMMUNICABLE, CONTAGIOUS, TRANSMISSIBLE DISEASES

An infectious disease is a disease due to a specific infectious agent or its toxic products that arises through transmission of that agent or its products from an infected person, animal, or reservoir to a susceptible host, either directly or indirectly through an intermediate plant or animal host, vector, or the inanimate environment. Infectious diseases are caused by an infectious agent, such as helminth, protozoa, fungus, bacteria, virus, or prion. Sometimes infectious agents are referred to as microorganisms, although helminths are really not microorganisms.

The term communicable disease is specific to those diseases that can be transmitted from an infected individual to another one directly or indirectly. It is sometimes used interchangeably for infectious diseases. Sometimes communicable diseases are defined as a subset of infectious diseases that can spread from person to person. Transmission can be either direct from other infected humans or indirect through vectors, airborne particles or vehicles.

Vectors are insects or animals that carry the infectious agent from person to person. Vehicles are contaminated objects or elements of the environment such as clothes, cutlery, water, milk, food, blood, plasma, parenteral solutions, or surgical instruments.

The term transmissible or contagious disease is often synonymous to communicable disease.

CHARACTERISTICS OF COMMUNICABLE DISEASES

Every communicable disease has a specific infectious agent or pathogen. Important aspects of these diseases are communicability, epidemicity, and immunity.

The dynamic of an epidemic is determined by the characteristics of its agent, its pattern of transmission, and by the susceptibility of its human hosts. The three main groups of pathogenic agents, bacteria, viruses and parasites, act very differently in this respect. A limited number of these agents cause most epidemics, and a thorough understanding of their biology has improved specific prevention measures. Vaccines, the most effective means of preventing communicable diseases, have been developed so far only for some viral and bacterial diseases. Vaccines work on both an individual basis, by preventing or attenuating clinical disease in a person exposed to the pathogen, and also on a population basis, by affecting herd immunity.

In a contagious, or propagated, epidemic, disease is passed from person to person, and the initial rise in the number of cases is gradual. The number of susceptible individuals and the potential sources of infection are the major factors determining the spread of disease. For example, Severe Acute Respiratory Syndrome (SARS) was first recognized as a global threat in March 2003. It spread rapidly to 26 countries, affecting adult men and women, with a fifth of all cases occurring among health-care workers.

THE GLOBAL BURDEN OF COMMUNICABLE DISEASES

Communicable diseases are a major cause of human suffering in terms of both morbidity and mortality throughout human history. The spread of communicable diseases was affected by various steps in human civilization. For example, parasitic and zoonotic diseases have become more common after domestication of animals, airborne viral and bacterial infections after large settlements and urbanization. Throughout the ages, humanity suffered from large pandemics such as plague, smallpox, cholera, and influenza but also from the more silent killers of chronic communicable diseases such as tuberculosis and syphilis.

Although there have been many advances in the prevention and treatment of communicable diseases, they remain significant causes of morbidity and mortality for the world's population in developed as well as developing countries. Morbidity due to communicable diseases is very common in spite of the progress accomplished in recent decades.

World Health Statistics 2016 indicate:

- In 2014, the global human immunodeficiency virus (HIV) incidence rate among adults aged 15–49 years was 0.5 per 1000 uninfected population, with 2 million people becoming infected. HIV incidence was highest in the WHO African Region at 2.6 per 1000 uninfected population in 2014, as compared with other WHO regions where incidence among adults aged 15–49 years ranged from 0.1 to 0.4

per 1000 uninfected.

- In 2014, there were 9.6 million new tuberculosis (TB) cases (133 per 100 000 population) and 1.5 million TB deaths, including 0.4 million deaths among HIV-positive people. In 2014, the largest number of new TB cases occurred in the WHO South-East Asia Region and WHO Western Pacific Region, accounting for 58% of new cases globally. However, Africa carried the most severe burden, with 281 cases per 100 000 population.

- In 2015, the malaria incidence rate was 91 per 1000 persons at risk, with an estimated 214 million cases and 438 000 deaths (more than two thirds of which occurred in children under 5 years of age). Sub-Saharan Africa has the highest burden, with an incidence rate of 246 per 1000 persons at risk, accounting for roughly 90% of all cases and deaths globally.

- For viral hepatitis no estimates of incidence are available yet. Global coverage of infants receiving three doses of hepatitis B vaccination was 82% in 2014.

- In 2014, at least 1.7 billion people in 185 countries required mass or individual treatment and care for neglected tropical diseases (NTDs).

The risk of acquiring infectious diseases varies greatly depending on socioeconomic determinants such as poverty and housing conditions, sex (for example, in the case of HIV infection in women, and tuberculosis in men) and environmental conditions which are influenced by different factors, including climate. In 2012, an estimated 871 000 deaths (mostly from infectious diseases) were caused by the contamination of drinking-water, bodies of water (such as rivers and reservoirs) and soil, and by inadequate hand-washing facilities and practices resulting from inadequate or inappropriate services. Almost half (45%) of these deaths occurred in the WHO African Region, where 13% of the global population lived.

EMERGING AND RE-EMERGING INFECTIONS

Emerging infections can be defined as infections that have recently appeared within a population or that may have existed before but are rapidly increasing their geographic range and prevalence. They may be further classified as newly-emerging infections, re-emerging infections, or deliberately emerging infections.

Over the past three decades, more than 40 new pathogens have been identified, some of them with global importance: Bartonella henselae, Borrelia burgdorferi, Campylobacter, Cryptosporidium, Cyclospora, Ebola virus, Escherichia coli O157:H7, Ehrlichia, Hantaan virus, Helicobacter, Hendra virus, Hepatitis C and E, HIV, HTLV-I and II, Human herpes virus 6 and 8, Human metapneumovirus, Legionella, new variant Creutzfeldt-Jakob disease agent, Nipah virus, Norovirus, Parvovirus B19, Rotavirus, SARS Coronavirus, etc.

Of these, HIV has had the greatest impact. Other examples include Ebola virus, Marburg virus, Crimean-Congo haemorrhagic fevers virus, West Nile virus, dengue virus, SARS coronavirus, and new variants of influenza A. A small epidemic of new variant Creutzfeldt–Jakob disease (a prion disease) in humans followed an epidemic of bovine spongiform encephalopathy in cattle. Also, development of antibiotic resistance has led to new outbreaks of familiar bacteria, including multidrug resistant (MDR) tuberculosis and methicillin resistant staphylococcus aureus (MRSA).

While some of these emerging diseases appear to be genuinely new, others, such as viral haemorrhagic fever, may have existed for centuries yet were recognized only recently because ecological or other environmental changes have increased the risk of human infection, or because the ability to detect such infections has improved. Changes in hosts, agents and environmental conditions are thought to be responsible for epidemics like those from diphtheria, syphilis and gonorrhea that occurred in the early 1990s in the newly independent states of Eastern Europe.

Influenza pandemics arise when a novel influenza virus emerges, infects humans and spreads efficiently among them. The virus of most recent concern is the H5N1 strain of influenza A, one of many viruses that usually infect poultry and migratory birds. Severe influenza pandemics in 1918, 1957 and 1968 caused the deaths of tens of millions of people; for example, between 40 million and 50 million people died in the 1918 pandemic. Based on projections from the 1957 pandemic, between 1 million and 4 million human deaths could occur if the H5N1 virus mutates to cause a readily transmissible form of human influenza.

IMPORTANCE OF COMMUNICABLE DISEASE EPIDEMIOLOGY

Epidemiology developed from the study of outbreaks of communicable disease and of the interaction between agents, hosts, vectors and reservoirs. The ability to describe the circumstances that tend to spark epidemics in human populations – war, migration, famine and natural disasters – has increased our ability to control the spread of communicable disease through surveillance, prevention, quarantine and treatment.

A complete understanding of the causative agent and transmission is always useful but not absolutely necessary. The most famous example is that of John Snow, who linked cholera transmission to water contamination during the London cholera epidemic of 1854 by comparing deaths from those households served by the Southward & Vauxhall Company with those served by another water company. John Snow further confirmed his hypothesis that the disease was spread by contaminated water by the observation that the cases of disease in the Broad Street area diminished after the handle of the pump serving the area was removed.

ETIOLOGY OF COMMUNICABLE DISEASE

Communicable diseases occur as a result of the interaction among:

- the infectious agent or **pathogen**
- the **host**
- the environment

This epidemiologic triangle recognizes three major factors---agent, host, and environment---in the pathogenesis of disease. This model is particularly well suited to an explanation of the etiology of communicable diseases, and current concepts of the etiology of communicable diseases have used this triad to construct more complex multivariate models of causality. In this section, we will consider how agent, host, and environment relate to the key topics in communicable disease epidemiology.

INFECTIOUS AGENT OR PATHOGEN

Infection is the entry and development or multiplication of an infectious agent in the host. Infection is not equivalent to disease, as some infections do not produce clinical disease. The specific characteristics of each agent are important in determining the nature of the infection, which is determined by such factors as:

Infectivity: Infectivity refers to the capacity of the pathogen to enter and multiply in a susceptible host and thus produce infection or disease. Polio and measles are diseases of high infectivity. The secondary attack rate is an indicator of infectivity.

Pathogenicity: Pathogenicity refers to the capacity of the pathogen to cause disease in the infected host, as measured by the ratio of the number of persons developing clinical illness to the number infected. Measles is a disease of high pathogenicity (few subclinical cases), whereas polio is a disease of low pathogenicity (most cases of polio are subclinical).

Virulence: Virulence refers to the severity of the disease, which can vary from very low to very high. The rabies virus, which virtually always produces fatal disease in humans, is an extremely virulent agent. Once a virus has been attenuated in a laboratory and is of low virulence, it can be used for immunization, as with the poliomyelitis virus. A measure of virulence is the proportion of total cases that are severe. If the disease can be fatal, virulence is reflected by the case fatality rate (CFR).

Toxigenicity: Toxigenicity refers to the capacity of the pathogen to produce a toxin or poison. The pathologic effects of diseases such as botulism and shellfish poisoning result from the toxin produced by the causative microorganism rather than from the microorganism itself.

Antigenicity and Immunogenicity: Antigenicity refers to the ability of the pathogen to induce antibody production in the host. A related term is immunogenicity, which refers to an infection's ability to produce specific immunity. Agents may or may not induce long-term immunity against infection. For example, repeated reinfection is common with gonococci, whereas reinfection with measles virus is rare.

Variability: Variability of the pathogen refers to antigen variation, virulence variation, drug resistance variation and parasite-host variation.

HOST

The host is the second link in the chain of infection and is defined as the person or animal that provides a suitable place for an infectious agent to grow and multiply under natural conditions.

Exposure to infectious disease agents depends on both intrinsic (internal) and extrinsic (external) host factors. Extrinsic host factors are the method of transmission of the microorganism as well as the host behavior. Exposure to microorganisms which are transmitted by droplet or airborne modes is very common. Anyone who is out in the public is likely to be exposed to these microorganisms. Microorganisms which are transmitted by vectors result usually from special occupations or special settings (hobbies or leisure activities). For example, persons who love to be outdoors (camping, hiking, or working on fields or in the forest) are more likely to be bitten by ticks or mosquitoes and therefore more likely to develop one of the zoonotic diseases which are transmitted by these arthropods. Exposure to sexually transmitted microorganisms depends entirely on the sexual activities, number of sex partners, and/or lifestyle of the hosts and the carriers of these diseases.

The transmission of infectious diseases is also regulated by intrinsic factors that influence the host response. It depends on how many microorganisms are transmitted (dose), how virulent the strain is, and how the microorganisms enter the human body. The person's age at time of infection is important, too. In general, the probability of clinical disease increases with age (e.g., polio, Hepatitis). Preexisting level of immunity to the disease, the nutritional status of the host, as well as any preexisting disease will influence a successful transmission as well. Individuals with impaired immune response (HIV, patients on immunosuppressive therapy for cancer or transplant) have a higher risk of developing severe disease. Also personal habits or lifestyle factors such as smoking, drinking alcohol, drug abuse, or exercise can influence the host response. Smoking depresses the ciliary function of the bronchial tree and increases susceptibility to infections (e.g., tuberculosis). Alcohol consumption increases the risk for chronic Hepatitis infections. Also psychological factors such as motivation and attitude toward disease can contribute to the transmission of infectious disease agents.

ENVIRONMENT

The environment plays a critical role in the development of infectious diseases. The environment refers to the domain in which the disease-causing agent may exist, survive, or originate.

There are several factors which influence the spread of microorganisms in the environment. The spread of infectious diseases depends on:

1. The stability of the microorganism in the physical environment required for its transmission including resistance to desiccation, high or low temperature, and ultraviolet light

2. The number of microorganisms in the vehicle of transmission

3. The virulence and infectivity of the microorganisms

4. The availability of the proper vector or medium for the transmission

Environmental characteristics play a role on different levels:

1. Survival of the virus in the environment

2. Influence on the route of transmission

3. Influence on the behavior of the host

A warm environment enhances the transmission

of microorganisms transmitted by water. In tropical and temperate areas, summer increases contacts between humans and surface water. Summer brings more people outside, particularly in the evening, and increases contacts between humans and mosquitoes and other arthropod vectors.

In the cooler seasons in temperate climates, in the rainy season in tropical climates, people tend to stay and congregate indoors promoting transmission by air-borne or droplet mechanisms. Long stays in the hot and dry environment indoors impair the protective mechanisms of human mucous membranes and may facilitate the attachment of viruses onto the upper respiratory mucous membranes. The incidence of upper respiratory infections is as high in the middle of winter in the temperate climates as in the middle of the monsoon or rainy season in the tropical climates.

INFECTIOUS PROCESS & SPECTRUM OF COMMUNICABLE DISEASE

The **infectious process** may be broken down into the following steps. If the infectious disease agent does not gain a foothold, the person was only exposed and the infectious disease process ends. If the disease agent gains a foothold but no reaction is occurring, the person will be colonized but not infected. An infection occurs when the disease agent attaches itself to the epithelium and begins to multiply. The infectious disease agent will release cytotoxins which will damage the cells and injure the tissue which leads to the dissemination through the human body. Even after dissemination, humans might not show any signs and symptoms and are therefore considered asymptomatic or show clinical signs and symptoms and are then considered symptomatic.

Exposed means that a person is placed in a situation where effective transmission of an infectious agent could occur. Being exposed does not always mean that transmission did occur. For example, being in the same room as an infectious tuberculous patient is being exposed since tuberculosis is trans-

mitted by droplet nuclei. However, being in the same room with a person with HIV does not meet the criteria for exposure because conditions are not met for transmission to occur.

COLONIZATION AND INFESTATION

Not all exposures to agents lead to illness, and the full spectrum of disease in the community setting may involve much more than individuals presenting with clinical symptoms. Colonization refers to the situation where an infectious agent may multiply on the surface of the body without invoking tissue or immune response. Infestation describes the presence of a living infectious agent on the body's exterior surface, where a localized reaction may be invoked.

INFECTION SPECTRUM

The host, after exposure to an infectious agent, may progress through a chain of events leading from subclinical (inapparent) infection to an active case of the disease. The end result may be complete recovery, permanent disability, disfigurement, or death. For example, the common cold is usually self-limited, and a complete recovery can be expected. Smallpox at one time was greatly feared because of its high morbidity and mortality. A small proportion of untreated cases of Group A streptococcal infection (β hemolytic) may produce the incapacitating sequelae of rheumatic fever and nephritis.

Inapparent Infection: A subclinical or inapparent infection is one that has not yet penetrated the clinical horizon (i.e., does not have clinically obvious symptoms). Nevertheless, it is of epidemiologic significance because asymptomatic individuals could transmit the disease to other susceptible hosts. Isolation of infected individuals is more likely to occur when the infectious disease is clinically apparent (i.e., when the ratio of apparent to inapparent cases is high). To determine whether an infection has taken place in both symptomatic and asymptomatic individuals, one may search for serologic evidence of infection. An elevated blood antibody level suggests previous exposure and infection by the disease agent. For example, hepatitis A (infectious hepatitis) often is manifested as a subclinical infection in nursery school children, who may transmit the disease even though they do not have clinical symptoms. The infectious process may be tracked by monitoring blood antibody and enzyme responses following exposure, thus allowing epidemiologists and clinicians to determine whether infection has occurred.

The Iceberg phenomenon of infection: The iceberg phenomenon of infection is the idea that active clinical disease may represent the tip of an iceberg, with only a small proportion of infections and exposures to disease agents being apparent.

THREE LINKS IN EPIDEMIC PROCESS

The **epidemic process** of communicable diseases is different from the infectious process and refers to the development and spread of communicable disease in a population, rather than within an individual. Three important links in the process are the source of infection, the route of transmission and the susceptible population.

SOURCE OF INFECTION

The natural habitat of infectious agents, from which the host acquires infection, may include humans, animals and environmental sources. Knowledge of both the reservoir and the source of infection are necessary for implementing effective control measures. An important **source of infection** may be a carrier – an infected person who shows no evidence of clinical disease. The duration of the carrier state varies between agents. Carriers can be asymptomatic throughout the course of infection, or the carrier state may be limited to a particular phase of the disease. Carriers played a large role in the worldwide spread of the human immunodeficiency virus due to inadvertent sexual transmission during the long asymptomatic period.

Incubation period: The incubation period is the time interval between exposure to an infectious agent and the appearance of the first signs or symptoms of disease. During this interval, the infectious organism replicates within the host. The incubation period is often a relatively narrowly-defined period of hours,

days, or weeks for each disease agent, and provides a clue to the time and circumstance of exposure to the agent. It is common practice for the epidemiologist to take into account the incubation period when attempting to determine the source of an infectious disease outbreak. For example, the incubation period for a measles rash to appear is usually 10 days, but it ranges from 7 to 18 days. Another example is outbreaks of food-borne disease in which the incubation period helps epidemiologists determine the etiologic agent.

Infectious or communicability period: The infectious (infectivity) period is the length of time a person may transmit a microorganism. There are several patterns for infectious periods:

Short period at the end of the incubation period and at the beginning of the disease (measles, chickenpox)

Short period and a few individuals become chronic carriers (Hepatitis B)

Throughout the disease (open cases of active pulmonary tuberculosis, malaria).

Measuring infectivity is difficult. It is often the interpretation of observational studies on the occurrence of secondary cases. Factors such as amount of infectious agents put out by the source, closeness, length of contact, and susceptibility of the target contacts have to be considered. In recent times, nucleic acid testing has been used to find remnants of infectious disease agents in human or environmental materials, but their significance to transmission is difficult to interpret.

Some diseases have only humans as the reservoir; notable among these is smallpox, which has been successfully eradicated because the virus apparently does not survive outside the human reservoir. Other disease, such as typhoid fever, may induce a chronic carrier state in some individuals who are not symptomatic for the disease but can transmit it to other susceptible individuals. A famous case was Typhoid Mary, a New York City area cook in the early 20th century who was a notorious and unwitting typhoid carrier.

A source of infection is the actual person, animal,

or object from which the infection was acquired.

A source of contamination is the person, animal, or object from which environmental media are contaminated. For example, the cook is the source of contamination of the potato salad.

A vehicle is an inanimate object which serves to communicate disease, for example, a glass of water containing microbes or a dirty rag.

A vector is a live organism that serves to communicate disease. Best known examples are Anopheles mosquitoes and malaria as well as Ixodes ticks and Lyme disease.

ROUTE OF TRANSMISSION

The second link in the chain of infection is the transmission or spread of an infectious agent through the environment or to another person. Transmission may be direct or indirect (Table 12-1).

Table 12-1 Modes of transmission of an infectious agent

Direct transmission	Indirect transmission
Touching	Vehicle-borne (contaminated food, water, towels, farm tools, etc.)
Kissing	Vector-borne (insects, animals)
Sexual intercourse	Airborne, long-distance (dust, droplets)
Other contact (e.g. childbirth, medical procedures, injection of drugs, breastfeeding)	Parenteral (injections with contaminated syringes)
Airborne, short-distance (via droplets, coughing, sneezing)	
Transfusion (blood)	
Transplacental	

Direct contact transmission: Direct contact transmission results from a direct body surface to body surface contact and physical transfer of microorganisms. Direct contact occurs when shaking hands, taking pulse, turning a patient over, and having sexual intercourse. Blood transfusions and transplacental infection from mother to fetus are other important means of direct transmission.

Indirect contact transmission: Indirect contact

transmission may be vehicle-borne, vector-borne or airborne. Vehicle-borne transmission occurs through contaminated materials such as food, clothes, bedding and cooking utensils. Vector-borne transmission occurs when the agent is carried by an insect or animal (the vector) to a susceptible host; the agent may or may not multiply in the vector. Long-distance airborne transmission occurs when there is dissemination of very small droplets to a suitable point of entry, usually the respiratory tract. Dust particles also facilitate airborne transmission, for example, of fungal spores.

It is important to distinguish between types of transmission when selecting control methods. **Direct transmission** can be interrupted by preventing contact with the source; **indirect transmission** requires different approaches, such as the provision of mosquito nets, adequate ventilation, cold storage for foods or sterile syringes and needles.

Categories of Communicable Diseases by Route of Transmission

Air-borne/droplet transmission diseases: Tuberculosis is spread primarily by inhalation of airborne droplets produced through coughing or speaking and is a significant cause of morbidity and mortality throughout the world. Tuberculosis had become uncommon in many developed countries, including the United States, but beginning in the late 1990s it began to increase in frequency. Reasons for the resurgence include the increasing prevalence of human immunodeficiency virus infection, an increase in the homeless population, and importation of cases from endemic areas.

Food-borne diseases: Food-borne diseases are caused by agents that enter the body through the consumption of food or beverages. Most cases are caused by microorganisms, including bacteria, viruses, and parasites. Other agents such as the agent causing BSE (bovine spongiform encephalopathy, also known as "mad cow disease"), appear to be transmissible through the consumption of tainted beef.

Many cases of food-borne illness are not

reported, so it is impossible to get an exact count of the incidence of food-borne illness. The incidence of food-borne diseases is believed to be much higher in developing countries, where more than a million people die from diarrheal diseases every year. Outbreaks of food-borne illness occur in both developing and industrialized countries and can affect large numbers of people. For instance, an outbreak of hepatitis A in China in 1998, caused by consumption of contaminated clams, affected more than 300,000 individuals, and an outbreak of salmonellosis in the United States in 1994, caused by consumption of contaminated ice-cream, affected 224,000 people.

Water-borne diseases: In the past 150 years, much progress has been made in understanding and preventing the transmission of infectious water-borne diseases. Even so, water-borne pathogens continue to be transmitted to humans via recreational water contact and contaminated drinking water supplies throughout the world, resulting in morbidity and mortality that is preventable. Infections that result from contact with water-borne pathogens can result in either endemic or epidemic disease. Most water-borne diseases are endemic in a population—there is some baseline level of disease that occurs normally in a population. An epidemic is defined when cases occur in excess of the normal occurrence for that population. The elderly and immunocompromised populations are also at an increased risk for water-borne infections.

Cholera is an example of a water-borne disease. It is characterized as an acute enteric disease with sudden onset of diarrhea, vomiting, rapid dehydration, acidosis, and circulatory collapse. Caused by the bacterial agent Vibrio cholerae, it still occurs in many parts of the developing world. In the mid-1800s, physician John Snow recommended removal of the handle from a water pump in a London neighborhood, ending an outbreak of cholera that had killed more than 500 people in a 10-day period.

Blood-borne diseases: Blood-borne diseases are caused by pathogens such as viruses or bacteria that can be spread through contamination by blood and other body fluids. The most common blood-borne

diseases are hepatitis B, hepatitis C, and HIV/AIDS. Sporadic outbreaks of hemorrhagic fevers, such as Ebola, have been documented in Africa and other parts of the world since 1976. Common routes of infection with blood-borne diseases include unprotected sexual activity, contact with blood through needles or other sharps, and transmission from mother to child during the birth process.

Sexually transmitted diseases: Sexually transmitted diseases (STDs), also commonly referred to as sexually transmitted infections (STIs), are primarily spread through the exchange of bodily fluids during sexual contact. STDs may also be transmitted through blood-to-blood contact and from a woman to her baby during pregnancy or delivery (congenital transmission). Exposure to STDs can occur through any close exposure to the genitals, rectum, or mouth. Unprotected sexual contact increases the likelihood of contracting an STD. Abstaining from sexual contact can prevent STDs, and correct and consistent use of latex condoms reduces the risk of transmission. Important STDs include gonorrhea, chlamydia, genital herpes, syphilis, human papillomavirus or genital warts, lymphogranuloma venereum, trichomoniasis, bacterial vaginosis, human immunodeficiency virus (HIV, the cause of AIDS), and hepatitis B. Other infections that may be sexually transmitted include hepatitis C, cytomegalovirus, scabies, and pubic lice. Persons with an STD are at increased risk of HIV. Successful treatment of an STD cures the infection, resolves the clinical symptoms, and prevents transmission to others. Most STDs can be treated and cured, although important exceptions include HIV and genital herpes. HIV can be effectively managed with antiviral agents but is not currently curable and can cause death. Genital herpes is a recurrent, life-long infection, although symptoms may be managed.

STDs remain a major public health concern due to their physical and psychological effects, as well as their economic toll. The acquired immunodeficiency syndrome (AIDS) epidemic, has had especially severe consequences for the economic activities and health resources of many nations. Women, especially young women, ethnic minorities, and men who have sex with men (MSM) are often most affected by STDs including HIV-AIDS.

Vector-borne diseases: Vector-borne diseases are caused by infectious agents such as bacteria, viruses, or parasites that are transmitted to humans by vectors. In most instances, vectors are bloodsucking invertebrates, such as ticks, mosquitoes, flies, and other arthropods, although vertebrates, including rodents, raccoons, and dogs, can also be vectors of human disease. Infectious agents are most often transmitted by the bite, sting, or touch of a vector, but ingesting or handling the feces, urine, or other substances of an infected animal can also result in disease transmission. Vector-borne diseases are most common in tropical and subtropical regions where optimal temperatures and moisture levels promote the reproduction of arthropods, especially mosquitoes. Diseases such as malaria, dengue, sleeping sickness, and encephalitis are still present at endemic or epidemic levels in some parts of the world. Re-emergence of vector-borne disease is a constant concern due to the rapid rate at which they can spread. These diseases have played a large role in integrating public health agencies, research, and relief and assistance to areas that are troubled by vector-borne pathogens.

Insect-borne diseases: The war between humans and insects predates recorded history. Not only have insects played an adversarial role in human development by destroying crops and killing livestock, they are also vectors for viruses, bacteria, and parasites that infect and cause illness in humans. Insect-borne diseases affect population rates, trade, travel, and productivity. While the true impact on the global economy is incalculable, the cost is most likely billions and billions of dollars annually. Insects are on every continent, and consequently so are the diseases they carry. The incidence rates of many insect-borne diseases have decreased due to improved public health initiatives undertaken by both governmental and nongovernmental organizations. Unfortunately, such efforts must confront the amazing adaptability of both insects and pathogens.

Arbovirus diseases: Diseases transmitted by insects and other arthropods are mostly arboviral diseases. These are a diverse group of diseases that involve transmission of arboviruses between vertebrate hosts (for example, from animal to animal or from animal to human) by blood-feeding arthropod vectors. Examples of these vectors are sand flies, ticks, and mosquitoes, the last of which are responsible for transmission of the encephalitis virus. Enzootic (referring to diseases that afflict animals in a particular locality) viral activity was reported in 1992; viral isolates or antigens of arboviruses were found in wild birds, sentinel birds, and captured mosquitoes; epizootic cases were documented in horses.

Zoonotic diseases: Infectious diseases of humans can be divided into those that are communicable only between humans and those that are communicable to humans by nonhuman vertebrates (with backbones such as mammals, birds, reptiles, amphibians, and fish, referred to in this entry simply as "animals"). Infectious diseases that have vertebrate animal reservoirs and are potentially transmissible to humans under natural conditions are called zoonoses. Zoonotic diseases may be either enzootic (similar to endemic in human diseases) or epizootic (similar to epidemic in human diseases). Examples are rabies and plague. Because of the large number of domestic and wild animals that can serve as a source of zoonotic diseases, and the numerous means of transmission including vectors, bites, etc., zoonotic disease are often difficult to control. Public health veterinarians have a critical role in zoonotic disease surveillance, prevention, and control, but risk reduction increasingly requires application of multidisciplinary teams and a unified concept of medicine across human and animal species lines.

SUSCEPTIBLE POPULATION

Herd immunity: The term herd immunity refers to the immunity of a population, group, or community against an infectious disease when a large proportion of individuals are immune (through either vaccinations or past infections). Herd immunity can prevent the spread of a disease to unimmunized individuals; herd immunity confers protection to the population even though not every single individual has been immunized. For example, herd immunity against rubella may require that 85% to 90% of community residents are immune; for diphtheria it may be only 70%.

Individual immunity: Individual immunity includes nonspecific defense and disease-specific defense.

The human body is equipped with a number of means to reduce the likelihood that an agent will penetrate and cause disease. Most environmental agents are unable to enter the body because of the protective barrier afforded by our skin. Similarly, the mucosal surfaces also afford protection against foreign invaders. Tears and saliva can wash away would-be infectious agents. The low pH of our gastric juices is lethal to many agents that manage to enter the body via ingestion. The immune system is also highly developed to ingest, via phagocytes and macrophages, infectious agents.

Disease-specific defenses include immunity against a particular agent. Immunity refers to the resistance of the host to a disease agent and may be natural or artificial, active or passive.

Natural active immunity: This type of immunity results from an infection by the agent. For example, a patient develops long-term immunity to measles because of a naturally acquired infection.

Natural passive immunity: Preformed antibodies during pregnancy are transferred across the placenta to the fetal bloodstream to produce short-term immunity in the newborn.

Artificial active immunity: All or part of a microorganism or a modified part of that microorganism is administered to invoke an immunologic response. The response mimics the natural infection but presents little or no risk to the recipient. This type of immunity usually results from an injection with a vaccine that stimulates antibody production in the host.

Artificial passive immunity: Preformed antibody is administered to a recipient; the immunity is usually of short duration (half-life, 3 to 4 weeks) for immune globulin (gamma globulin) derived from the pooled plasma of adults. An example is prophylaxis against hepatitis A for individuals at risk.

PREVENTION AND CONTROL MEASURES FOR COMMUNICABLE DISEASES

Prevention of communicable diseases involves protective measures aimed at populations potentially under threat from environmentally-caused infectious diseases, insect vectors, or animals containing pathogens, in order to prevent an epidemic.

HEALTH EDUCATION

Having unhealthy habits and an unhealthy life-style is one of the main reasons for the eruption of epidemics of communicable diseases. Therefore, health education is an important weapon and resource for disease control and prevention. It can increase health knowledge and capability for self-care, and nurture better health habits and is a cost-effective policy.

IMPROVEMENT OF SANITARY CONDITIONS

Transmission of most communicable diseases is related to environmental sanitation and food hygiene. Therefore, it is fundamental for prevention and control of communicable diseases to improve sanitation systems in both the city and countryside, to keep drinking water clean, to strengthen food sanitation inspection, to enforce decontamination, and to improve the management of filth and human excreta.

ENHANCE SURVEILLANCE OF COMMUNICABLE DISEASES

Surveillance of communicable diseases includes recording cases and deaths from communicable diseases, and by describing the species, characteristics, and geographic distributions of various pathogen, their vectors, and animal hosts. It also includes monitoring population levels of immunity and immunization status.

Reports of notifiable communicable diseases provide the main measures of surveillance, control, and eradication of communicable diseases in China. The reporting process requires rapidity, thoroughness, and accuracy, so that agencies of disease prevention and control are able to understand the epidemic situation in time and make good decisions with regards to the strategy and measures to control and eliminate diseases.

In China, notifiable diseases are grouped into A, B, and C categories and include 39 communicable diseases as of the end of 2014. The types of communicable diseases reported may increase or decrease or change according to the epidemic situation.

Category A, 2 conditions: plague and cholera.

Category B, 26 conditions: SARS, AIDS, viral hepatitis, poliomyelitis, human highly pathogenic avian influenza, measles, epidemic hemorrhagic fever, rabies, epidemic encephalitis type B, dengue fever, anthrax, bacillary dysentery and intestinal amoebiasis, pulmonary tuberculosis, typhoid and paratyphoid, epidemic cerebrospinal meningitis, pertussis, diphtheria, tetanus neonatorum, scarlet fever, brucellosis, gonorrhea, syphilis, schistosomiasis, malaria, and human H7N9 avian influenza.

Category C, 11 conditions: hand-foot-mouth disease, influenza (including H1N1 influenza), mumps, rubella, leprosy, acute hemorrhage conjunctivitis, epidemic and endemic typhus, black fever, echinococcosis, filariasis, and communicable diarrhea not due to cholera, bacillary dysentery, intestinal amoebiasis, typhoid, or paratyphoid.

TERRITORY HEALTH QUARANTINE

In order to prevent communicable diseases from being imported or exported, health quarantine stations are established along international borders at harbors, airports, and border towns to identify and treat ill passengers or crew and to inspect vehicles, goods, luggage, mail, and animals for pathogens. Currently, three communicable diseases require quarantine in China: plague, cholera, and yellow fever, with quarantine periods of 6 days, 5 days and 6 days, respectively. Other communicable diseases also require isolation in China, such as SARS, avian influenza, Ebola, etc.

VACCINATION

Vaccination is an artificial immunization method by which antigens or antibodies are inoculated into hosts, which makes human bodies acquires immunity against specific communicable diseases, so as to protect susceptible populations and prevent communicable diseases.

Types of vaccination

Active immunization: Immunogenic substances are inoculated into the human body to make the body produce a specific antibody. This active immunity measure should be taken a few weeks before exposure to the communicable disease, so that there is enough time to generate immunity. There are six types of reagents for active immunity, including live attenuated vaccine, inactivated vaccines, toxoid vaccines, component vaccines (subunit vaccines), genetically engineered vaccines, and compounded multivalent vaccines.

Passive immunization: Serum or a preparation containing an antibody is administered and provides specific immunity to the communicable disease immediately. The two types of reagents commonly used for passive immunization are immune serum and immunoglobulin (gamma globulin and globulin placentae).

Passive-active immunization: A set of reagents combines characteristics of both passive and active immunity, and they can be used for a few communicable diseases. For example, when blocking the maternal-infant transmission of hepatitis B virus, giving neonatal hepatitis B immune globulin (HBIG) and the whole hepatitis B vaccination.

Planned immunization

Planned immunization refers to vaccination of a population with scientific procedures determined according to information provided by disease surveillance about epidemic circumstances and population immunity levels against communicable diseases. The goal is to enhance population immunity levels, and to prevent, control, or eradicate corresponding communicable diseases. There are three prerequisites to putting planned vaccination into practice: ①supply enough qualified vaccines; ②ensure the transportation and storage of vaccines in a cold chain; ③achieve a high vaccination rate in the target population.

Immunization of children is currently the emphasis in China. For children under 7 years old, Bacille Calmette-Guerin (BCG) vaccine for tuberculosis, a trivalent vaccine for poliomyelitis, diphtheria-pertussis-tetanus toxoid vaccine, measles vaccine, and Hepatitis B vaccine are provided. Later booster immunization is given if necessary to ensure that Children acquire immunity to tuberculosis, poliomyelitis, whooping cough (pertussis), diphtheria, tetanus, measles and Hepatitis B.

Expanded program on immunization

WHO initiated the Expanded Program on Immunization (EPI) in 1974 to provide countries with guidance and support to improve vaccine delivery and to help make vaccines available for all children. China has participated in the EPI formally since 1981. National immunization programs in China are now responsible for improving access to the traditional EPI antigens and introducing new vaccines. Since 1992, Hepatitis B vaccine has been provided to all children. At present, an expanding national immunization programs is introducing vaccines against hepatitis A, epidemic cerebrospinal meningitis, encephalitis B, rubella, epidemic parotitis (mumps), epidemic hemorrhagic fever, anthrax, and leptospirosis (febris hebdomadis). In addition to delivering vaccinations, national immunization programs are concerned with ensuring the quality and safety of immunization through adoption of safe injection technologies and proper cold chain and vaccine stock maintenance.

MEASURES TO CONTROL SOURCES OF INFECTION

Patients

"Five earlies" must be met: early detection, early diagnosis, early reporting, early isolation, and early treatment. Management at different levels should be carried out for patients diagnosed with, or suspected of having, communicable diseases. Isolation of patients from surrounding susceptible populations is the most effective way to prevent the spread of pathogens. It helps to not only sterilize the site and manage the disease, but also to treat patients promptly. Therefore, isolation can play an important role in controlling and eliminating the infection source.

Carriers

Screening is undertaken using simple assays with high sensitivity and specificity to find pathogen carriers. For staff working in food industries and service sectors, physical examinations should be done before employment and periodically afterwards. Once pathogen carriers are found, they should not only get treatment, but should also be recorded and educated.

Exposures

Quarantine can be the key measure to reduce the risk of exposure. Quarantine periods are dependent upon the **incubation period** of the communicable disease. According to the type of disease and the immune status, different steps ought to be followed.

Isolated observation: Persons who have had contact with a source of communicable diseases of category A are confined to an assigned place to be observed, inspected, tested, and treated.

Medical observation: Persons who have had contact with a source of communicable diseases of category B and C may conduct their normal daily lives, but they need to have physical examinations, temperature measurements, inspections, and disinfection as necessary.

Emergency vaccination and drug prevention: Vaccination can be carried out on the contacts to induce immunity to the communicable diseases with long incubation periods, such as measles. In addition, antimicrobial drugs can be used for prevention.

Animal reservoirs: Different measures may be taken with regard to animal reservoirs according to their economic value and the type of disease. Any reservoir of animals posing a great potential danger should be killed and burned or buried deeply. Animals with economic value but posing only limited potential hazard can be isolated and treated. In addition, domestic animals and pets should be vaccinated and quarantined.

MEASURES TO INTERRUPT THE ROUTES OF TRANSMISSION

Different measures should be taken according to the range of the epidemic and route of transmission. The specific measures include disinfection and deinsectization programs.

Disinfection

Disinfection is a measure to eliminate pathogenic microorganisms from the environment using physical or chemical methods. It can be classified into prophylactic disinfection and disinfection of an epidemic focus.

Prophylactic disinfection: This disinfection method focuses on places or items that are possibly contaminated by communicable pathogens.

Disinfection of the epidemic focus: The epidemic focus where there are, or were, communicable pathogens is disinfected to eliminate the pathogens discharged from the sources of infection. This measure is divided into two types: current disinfection and terminal disinfection.

- Current disinfection is to concomitantly disinfect excrement, excreta, and other contaminated items when the source of infection exists in an epidemic focus.

- Terminal disinfection is a thorough disinfection of the epidemic focus after the communicable source has been removed (recovered, died, or left), so that any remaining pathogenic microorganisms are totally eliminated.

Deinsectization

Deinsectization is the method used to kill harmful insects, especially the vector-borne arthropods that transmit pathogens in the environment.

MEASURES FOR SUSCEPTIBLE POPULATION

Immunoprophylaxis: This term relates to measures that enhance the immunity level of the host and efficiently prevent the corresponding communicable disease. Immunoprophylaxis is the goal of planned immunization and one of the most important measures for control and elimination of communicable diseases. Epidemiological studies are useful to determine if the widespread use of vaccine has led to suppression of disease with continuation of circulation of the agent or to the total disappearance of the infectious agent.

Drug prophylaxis: For some communicable diseases for which a drug is available for prevention and treatment, drug prophylaxis may be prescribed for the high risk population.

Other protective measures: In epidemic seasons, protective measures such as insecticide-treated bed nets, face masks, gloves, leg guards, and condoms can be provided to the susceptible population to prevent infection.

SUMMARY

To prevent diseases, it is important to understand the causative agents, risk factors and circumstances that lead to a specific disease. This is especially important for communicable disease prevention, since simple interventions may break the chain of transmission. With the ultimate goal of control and eradication of communicable diseases, communicable disease epidemiology mainly involves studies of: (1) the etiology of communicable diseases, (2) the occurrence and transmission of communicable diseases in a population; (3) the natural and social factors that affect the transmission of communicable diseases; (4) preventive strategies and measures to block the transmission route and protect the susceptible population; and (5) the effectiveness of preventive and control strategies and measures.

Today the world is smaller than ever before, international travel and a worldwide food market make us all potentially vulnerable to communicable diseases, no matter where we live. Not only are etiologic agents changing, the world's population is changing as well. In non-industrialized countries, life expectancy is increasing and the elderly are more likely to acquire a chronic disease, such as cancer or diabetes, in their lifetime. Because of these conditions, or their treatment, older populations also have an increased susceptibility to infectious diseases and are more likely to develop life-threatening complications.

Knowledge of communicable disease epidemiology is expanding. While basic epidemiological methods and principles still apply today, improved laboratory diagnoses and techniques help to confirm cases faster and can show how cases are related to each other, thereby enabling health authorities to implement measures to prevent communicable diseases from spreading. Better computers can improve data analysis, and the internet allows access to in depth disease-specific information. Computer connectivity also improves disease reporting for surveillance purposes, and the epidemiologist can implement faster preventive measures and identify disease clusters and outbreaks more quickly. With all these changes, there is renewed emphasis on communicable disease epidemiology, and this makes it an exciting field to work in.

(Bei Wang)

 ## STUDY QUESTIONS

1. *Name the epidemic factors and characterize them briefly.*

2. *Name the phases of transmission of pathogenic microbes from one microorganism to another.*

3. *What major factors are involved in the transmission of pathogenic microorganisms?*

4. *What measures are necessary to control the source of infection and to disrupt the route of infection transmission?*

5. *What measures are taken to strengthen insusceptibility of population to infectious diseases?*

IMPORTANT TERMINOLOGY

communicable disease epidemiology	传染病流行病学
emerging infections	新发传染病
pathogen	病原体
host	宿主
infectious process	传染 / 感染过程
infection spectrum	感染谱
epidemic process	流行过程
source of infection	传染源
route of transmission	传播途径
susceptible population	易感人群
carrier	携带者
incubation period	潜伏期
direct transmission	直接传播
indirect transmission	间接传播
air-borne/droplets disease	空气 / 飞沫传播疾病
food-borne diseases	食源性疾病
water-borne diseases	介水传播疾病
blood-borne diseases	血液传播疾病
sexually transmitted diseases (STDs) / sexually transmitted infections (STIs)	性传播疾病 / 性传播感染
vector-borne diseases	虫媒传播疾病
zoonotic diseases	人畜共患病
herd immunity	群体免疫力
vaccination	免疫接种
quarantine	检疫（留验）

RECOMMENDED READING AND WEB SITE

1. www.who.int/en/
2. www.cdc.gov
3. www.chinacdc.cn
4. www.icdc.cn

REFERENCE

W. Ahrens, I. Pigeot. Handbook of Epidemiology.2nd ed.©Springer Science+Business Media, New York, 2014

R. Bonita, R. Beaglehole, T. Kjellström. Basic epidemiology. 2nd ed. World Health Organization. 2006

World health statistics 2016: monitoring health for the SDGs, sustainable development goals. © World Health Organization 2016.[E-ISBN 978 92 4 069569 6 (PDF)]

M. L. Volovaskaya. Epidemiology and Fundamentals of Infectious Diseases.

13 Noncommunicable Chronic Disease Epidemiology

Noncommunicable diseases (NCDs) are the major health Challenges of the 21st century. No government can afford to ignore the rising burden of NCDs. Cardiovascular diseases (CVDs), cancer, respiratory diseases and diabetes mellitus are the major NCDs that affect health and quality of life, but they can be effectively prevented and controlled.

OVERVIEW

Concept

Noncommunicable diseases (NCDs), also known as chronic diseases, are diseases that are not passed from person to person and have insidious onset, long duration and generally slow progression (usually longer than three months from the onset). The causes of NCDs are complex or uncertain. The four main types of NCDs are cardiovascular diseases (CVDs), cancer, chronic respiratory diseases and diabetes mellitus. These diseases are caused mainly by behavioral factors, lifestyle, environmental factors, occupational exposure or genetic factors.

NCD Burden

The burden of NCDs has been a major public health challenge that undermines social and economic development worldwide. A total of 56 million deaths occurred worldwide during 2012. Of these, 38 million were due to NCDs. Nearly three-quarters of NCD-related deaths occurred in low-and middle-income countries. The leading causes of NCD-related deaths in 2012 were CVDs (17.5 million deaths, or 46.2% of NCD deaths), cancer (8.2 million, or 21.7%

of NCD deaths), respiratory diseases including asthma and chronic obstructive pulmonary disease (COPD) (4.0 million, or 10.7% of NCD deaths) and diabetes (1.5 million, or 4% of NCD deaths).

In 2012, the age-standardized mortality rate for NCDs was $539/10^5$ globally, and this rate was lowest in high-income countries ($397/10^5$) and highest in low-income ($625/10^5$) and lower-middle-income countries ($673/10^5$). Figure13-1 shows the proportion of NCD-related deaths by cause in 2012 among people under 70 years of age. CVDs were responsible for the largest proportion of NCD-related deaths (37%), followed by cancers (27%) and chronic respiratory diseases (8%). Diabetes was responsible for 4% of deaths, and other NCDs accounted for approximately 24% of all NCD deaths.

NCDs are usually lifelong diseases that not only affect a patient's physical health but also reduce the quality of life and pose a heavy financial burden to individuals, families and society. The disability-adjusted life year (DALY) is a measure of overall disease burden expressed as the number of years lost due to ill health, disability or early death. The economic burden includes direct and indirect costs. The direct costs are medical costs related to the diagnosis and treatment of diseases including transportation, accommodation, food and outpatient and inpatient expenses. The indirect costs are calculated as a loss of income due to disease-related inability to work. During 2011-2025, the cumulative economic losses due to NCDs under a "business as usual" scenario in low-and middle-income countries have been estimated at US$ 7 trillion.

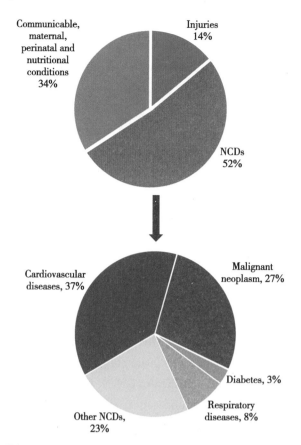

Figure 13-1. Proportion of global deaths in individuals under the age of 70 by cause of death, 2012. [from Global status report on noncommunicable diseases 2014].

Poverty and NCDs

A strong link exists between poverty and NCDs at the household level. In most countries, people with lower socioeconomic status are mostly at risk of developing NCDs and dying prematurely from these conditions. This may be because the poor population has a higher probability of exposure to risk factors. Also, the poor are less likely to benefit from early diagnosis and proper management, which may contribute to the higher prevalence and mortality of NCDs. The long-term course of illness posed by chronic diseases may prevent people from pursuing gainful employment, and the burden of the health care costs can result in catastrophic health expenditure.

NCD Trends

While the mortality of infectious disease has declined in recent decades, the number of NCD-related deaths has increased from 6.7 million in 2000 to 8.5 million in 2012 in the WHO South-East Asia Region and from 8.6 million to 10.9 million in the Western Pacific Region. Unlike infectious diseases, NCDs seldom occur as outbreaks or present short-term fluctuations, and therefore, people are more concerned about their long-term trends. It is expected that in the next 20 years, the annual global deaths from infectious diseases will be reduced by approximately 7 million, but the number of people who will die from CVDs will be increased by 6 million each year, and the number of cancer deaths will be increased by approximately 4 million. If the condition of "business as usual" continues, the annual number of deaths from NCDs will increase to 55 million by 2030. In Africa, NCDs have been projected to be on the rise which will exceed infectious, maternal, perinatal and nutritional diseases as the most common causes of death by 2030.

Population Distribution

A gender difference exists in the mortality of major NCDs, and this difference is obvious among countries. For example, in 2008, in low-and middle-income countries, the age-standardized mortality rate for NCDs was $756/10^5$ among men, which was significantly higher than that among women ($565/10^5$). Although NCDs mainly occur in adults, the exposure to risk factors usually begins in early life, and children are at a higher risk of dying from treatable NCDs such as rheumatic heart disease, type 1 diabetes, asthma and leukemia.

Geographic Distribution

The main causes of death are closely related to the development level of the country or region in which the patients live. In high-income countries, people mainly die of CVDs, COPD, cancer, diabetes and other NCDs. In low-income countries, most people die of infectious diseases, such as respiratory infections, diarrhea, HIV/AIDS, tuberculosis and malaria. It is noteworthy that the prevalence of NCDs in the African region is growing rapidly, although infectious diseases are still common in these areas.

INTRODUCTION TO THE MAJOR NCDS

Epidemiological evidence indicates that four major NCDs—CVDs (heart disease and stroke), cancer, chronic respiratory disease and diabetes—make the greatest contribution to the NCD burden.

CVDs

CVDs are caused by disorders of the heart and blood vessels, including coronary heart disease (heart attacks), cerebrovascular disease (stroke), hypertension, peripheral artery disease, rheumatic heart disease, congenital heart disease and heart failure. CVDs have been ranked as the primary cause of death globally. An estimated 17.5 million people died from CVDs in 2012, which represented 31% of all deaths. Among these deaths, 7.4 million were due to coronary heart disease, and 6.7 million were due to stroke. People living in low-and middle-income countries often benefit less from integrated primary health care services for early detection and intervention. As a result, many diseases are detected late in the course of illness, and patients die at younger ages from CVDs than they do from other NCDs, often during their most productive years. At least three-quarters of the world's deaths from CVDs occur in low-and middle-income countries. The poorest people are mostly affected by CVDs. At the household level, sufficient evidence is emerging to prove that CVDs and other NCDs contribute to poverty due to catastrophic health spending and high out-of-pocket expenditure. At the macroeconomic level, CVDs put a heavy burden on the economies of low-and middle-income countries.

The most important behavioral risk factors for CVDs are unhealthy diet, physical inactivity, tobacco use and harmful alcohol use. Cessation of tobacco use, reduction in dietary salt, consumption of fruits and vegetables, regular physical activity and avoiding harmful alcohol use have been shown to reduce the risk of CVDs. In addition, drug treatment for diabetes, hypertension and high blood lipids may reduce the risk of cardiovascular diseases and prevent heart attacks and strokes. It is essential to create a policy environment for making healthy choices affordable and available to motivate people to adopt healthy behaviors.

Cancer

The transformation from a normal cell into a tumor cell is a multistage process, typically in which a precancerous lesion progresses to a malignant tumor. These changes are the result of interactions among genetic factors and external agents, including physical, chemical and biological carcinogens. Cancer is a major cause of morbidity and mortality, with approximately 14 million new cases and 8 million cancer-related deaths in 2012. Among men, the five most common cancer sites in 2012 were the lung (16.7%), prostate (15.0%), colorectum (10.0%), stomach (8.5%) and liver (7.5%). Among women, the five most common cancer sites were the breast (25.2%), colorectum (9.2%), lung (8.7%), cervix (7.9%) and stomach (4.8%). Lung cancer had the highest incidence ($34.2/10^5$) and prostate cancer had the second highest incidence ($31.1/10^5$) among men. Breast cancer had a substantially higher incidence ($43.3/10^5$) followed by colorectal cancer ($14.3/10^5$) among women (Figure 13-2). Cancer is becoming the major cause of premature deaths among patients with NCDs. Approximately one-third of cancer deaths are due to the following five behavioral and dietary risks: high body mass index (BMI), low fruit and vegetable intake, lack of physical activity, tobacco smoking and harmful use of alcohol.

COPD

COPD is a lung ailment that is characterized by a persistent blockage of airflow from the lungs. It is a life-threatening disease that interferes with normal breathing. The most common symptoms of COPD are breathlessness, abnormal sputum and a chronic cough. Daily activities, such as walking up a short flight of stairs or carrying a suitcase, can become very difficult for patients with COPD as the condition gradually worsens.

More than 3 million people died of COPD in

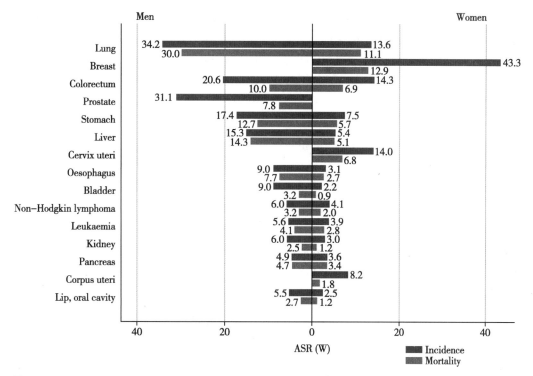

Figure 13-2. Estimated age-standardized cancer incidence and mortality rates (ASR) per 100,000, by major sites, in men and women, 2012. [from World Cancer Report 2014]

2012, representing 6% of all global deaths in that year. At one time, COPD was more common in men than in women, but as a result of increased tobacco use among women in high-income countries and the higher risk of exposure to indoor air pollution in low-income countries, the disease now affects men and women almost equally. More than 90% of COPD deaths occur in low-and middle-income countries where effective strategies for prevention and control are not always implemented or accessible.

The primary cause of COPD is tobacco smoking (including second-hand or passive exposure). Other risk factors include indoor air pollution (such as from solid fuel used for cooking and heating), outdoor air pollution, occupational dust and chemical exposure and frequent lower respiratory infections during childhood. COPD is not curable, but early interventions can help control symptoms and increase the quality of life for people with the illness.

Diabetes

Diabetes is a chronic disease that occurs either when the pancreas does not produce enough insulin or when the body cannot effectively use the insulin it

produces. There are three different types of diabetes: type 1, type 2 and gestational diabetes. The main symptoms of diabetes include increased thirst, more often than usual urination and increased hunger. Patients with diabetes often lack early intervention, proper treatment and diabetic medications, which results in multiple complications including neurological, vascular or visual disorders, heart disease, stroke, lower limb amputation, kidney failure and other chronic conditions. Adults with diabetes have a 2-to 3-fold increased risk of heart attacks and strokes. Combined with reduced blood flow, nerve damage in the feet increases the chance of foot ulcers. Diabetic retinopathy is an important cause of blindness and occurs as a result of long-term accumulated damage to the small blood vessels in the retina. It is estimated that 2.6% of global blindness can be attributed to diabetes.

The global prevalence of diabetes among adults over 18 years of age has risen from 4.7% in 1980 to 8.5% in 2014. The number of people living with diabetes has risen from 108 million in 1980 to 422 million in 2014. Diabetes can be managed, and its consequences can be avoided or delayed. Healthy diet, regular physical activity, maintenance of a normal body weight and avoidance of tobacco use are effective in preventing or delaying the onset of type 2 diabetes.

RISK FACTORS

The vast majority of NCDs are caused by a limited number of known and preventable risk factors, mainly including tobacco smoking, physical inactivity and an unhealthy diet. These behaviors contribute to elevated blood pressure (hypertension), blood sugar (diabetes), and blood lipids (dyslipidemia) as well as obesity. Social, political, economic and environmental factors also contribute to the rising NCD trends.

Tobacco Use

Tobacco contains approximately 4,000 chemicals, including at least 250 known species of harmful substances and more than 50 carcinogens. The tobacco epidemic is one of the biggest public health threats that the world has ever faced and kills approximately 6 million people annually. More than 5 million of those deaths are directly attributable to tobacco use. By 2020, this number will increase to 7.5 million and account for 10% of all deaths. Second-hand smoke is the smoke that fills restaurants, offices or other enclosed spaces when people burn tobacco. There is no safe level of exposure to second-hand tobacco smoke. More than 600,000 tobacco-related deaths are the result of non-smokers being exposed to the second-hand smoke.

Smoking is estimated to cause approximately 71% of lung cancer, 42% of chronic respiratory disease and nearly 10% of CVDs. In recent years, the amount of tobacco use has started to decrease in many high-income countries, but the consumption of tobacco in low-and middle-income countries has risen sharply. If this trend continues, by the year 2030, the deaths due to tobacco use will reach approximately 8 million, and 80% of premature deaths will occur in low-income countries.

Insufficient Physical Activity

Physical activity is any bodily movement produced by the skeletal muscles that uses energy, including sports, exercise and other activities, such as playing, walking, doing household chores, gardening or dancing. Compared with regular moderate-intensity physical activity, lack of exercise increases the risk of death by approximately 20%-30%. Each week, 150 minutes of moderate-intensity physical activity is estimated to reduce the risk of ischemic heart disease by 30%, diabetes by 27%, breast and colon cancer by 21%-25%.

Physical activity is a key factor in energy consumption and is very important to energy balance and weight control. Physical inactivity is the fourth leading risk factor for global mortality. Approximately 3.2 million people die each year due to physical inactivity. Regular physical activity can reduce the risk of CVDs including high blood pressure, diabetes, breast and colon cancer, and depression. Insufficient physical activity is highest in high-income countries but is now also seen in some middle-income countries, especially among women.

Increasing levels of physical activity can bring health benefits across age groups. Inactive people should start with small amounts of physical activity and gradually increase the duration, frequency and intensity over time. Both society and the general population can take action to increase physical activity. WHO member states have agreed to reduce physical inactivity by 10% by 2025 in the framework of the "Global Action Plan for the Prevention and Control of Noncommunicable Diseases 2013-2020".

Harmful Alcohol Use

Alcohol is a psychoactive substance with dependence-producing properties. It has been widely used for centuries and has impacted people and societies in many ways. The risk of alcohol is determined by the volume of alcohol consumed, the pattern of drinking and on rare occasions, the quality of alcohol. In 2010, it was estimated that the average alcohol consumption was 21.2 liters of pure alcohol for male drinkers and 8.9 liters for female drinkers.

Alcohol consumption is a causal factor for more than 200 diseases and injury conditions. Drinking alcohol is associated with the risk of developing health problems such as mental and behavioral disorders (for example, alcohol dependence), major NCDs, and unintentional and intentional injuries. In 2012, approximately 3.3 million global deaths (5.9% of all deaths) were attributable to alcohol consumption. Over half of these deaths occurred from NCDs, including cancers, CVDs and liver cirrhosis. A gender difference has been observed in alcohol-related mortality and morbidity. The percentage of alcohol-attributable deaths among men amounts to 7.6% of all global deaths compared with 4.0% of all deaths among women.

Unhealthy Diet

Unhealthy diets result in at least 14 million deaths per year, which represents 40% of all NCD-related deaths.

Fruit and vegetable consumption: Fruit and vegetable consumption is one element of a healthy diet. Fresh vegetables and fruits are important sources of vitamins, minerals, dietary fiber and phytochemicals. Approximately 16 million DALYs and 1.7 million deaths are attributable to low fruit and vegetable consumption worldwide each year. Adequate consumption of fruit and vegetables reduces the risk of CVDs, stomach cancer and colorectal cancer.

Salt intake: Dietary salt consumption is an important determinant of high blood pressure and overall CVD risk. Approximately 30% of high blood pressure can be attributed to excess intake. Intake of less than 5 grams of salt per person per day is recommended by the WHO. The Dietary Guidelines for Chinese Residents recommends 6 grams of salt per adult per day. However, data from various countries indicate that most populations are consuming much more salt than these recommended levels. It is estimated that decreasing dietary salt intake from the current global levels of 9-12 grams per day to the recommended level of 5 grams per day would have a major impact on blood pressure and CVDs.

Fat intake: Fat is an important source of human energy. It provides essential fatty acids and is beneficial to digestion and absorption of fat-soluble vita-

mins. However, excessive fat intake is a risk factor for obesity, raised cholesterol, atherosclerosis and other chronic diseases. Saturated fat intake can increase serum levels of total cholesterol (TC) and low-density lipoprotein cholesterol (LDLc). The trans-fatty acids can also increase the levels of LDLc and triglyceride (TG) and reduce high-density lipoprotein cholesterol (HDLc) levels. High consumption of saturated fats and trans-fatty acids is linked to heart disease, whereas unsaturated fatty acids from vegetable sources and polyunsaturated fatty acids can reduce the risk of type 2 diabetes.

Overweight and Obesity

Overweight and obesity are defined as abnormal or excessive fat accumulation that may impair health. The body mass index (BMI) is a simple index that is commonly used to classify overweight and obesity in adults. It is defined as a person's weight in kilograms divided by the height in meters squared (kg/m^2). The following subdivision (WHO, 1997) is used to classify BMIs: < 18.5 kg/m^2, underweight; 18.5 kg/m^2–24.9 kg/m^2: normal range; $>=25.0$ kg/m^2, overweight; and $>= 30.0$ kg/m^2, obese. The recommended criteria for overweight in Asian populations are $>= 23$ kg/m^2 and for obesity $>= 27$ kg/m^2. In 2014, more than 1.9 billion adults aged over 18 years were overweight. Of these, over 600 million adults were obese. In 2014, approximately 38% of men and 40% of women over 18 years of age were overweight, whereas 11% of men and 15% of women were obese. Overweight and obesity are major risk factors for CVDs (mainly heart disease and stroke), diabetes, musculoskeletal disorders (especially osteoarthritis), and some cancers (including endometrial, breast, ovarian, prostate, liver, gallbladder, kidney and colon cancer). The fundamental cause of overweight and obesity is an energy imbalance between calories consumed and expended.

Elevated Blood Pressure

High blood pressure changes the structure of the arteries. As a result, the risks for stroke, heart disease, kidney failure and other diseases increase with blood pressure. Elevated blood pressure is estimated to cause 7.5 million deaths worldwide, which accounts for 57 million DALYs. Globally, the overall prevalence of elevated blood pressure in adults aged 25 and over was approximately 40% in 2008. The proportion of the world's population with high blood pressure or uncontrolled hypertension fell modestly between 1980 and 2008. However, as a result of population growth and aging, the absolute number of people with uncontrolled hypertension rose from 600 million in 1980 to nearly 1 billion in 2008. Men have a slightly higher prevalence of raised blood pressure than do women, but this difference is only significant in some regions such as the United States and Europe.

Elevated Cholesterol

Consumption of foods with high saturated fat, physical inactivity and genetics can increase cholesterol levels. The levels of LDLs and HDLs are more important for health than TC. Because there is more information available about average TC levels in populations worldwide than about average LDLs and HDLs, researchers usually calculate the risk of elevated total blood cholesterol. Elevated TC is a major cause of disease burden in both developed and developing countries as a risk factor for ischemic heart disease and stroke. Globally, a third of ischemic heart disease is attributable to high cholesterol levels in the body. Overall, elevated cholesterol is estimated to cause 2.6 million deaths and 29.7 million DALYs annually. A 10% reduction in serum cholesterol in 40-year-old men has been reported to result in a 50% reduction in heart disease within 5 years. The same serum cholesterol reduction for 70-year-old men can result in an average 20% reduction in heart disease occurrence over the next 5 years.

Cancer-Associated Infections

Recent studies have found that some cancers are related to pathogens or chronic infectious diseases. At least 2 million cancer cases per year (18% of the global cancer burden) are attributable to a few specific chronic infections, and this fraction is substantially larger in low-income countries. The papillomavirus (HPV) is related to cervical cancer; hepatitis B and C virus are related to liver cancer; and helicobacter pylori (HP) is related to gastric cancer. These infections are largely preventable through vaccinations or measures to avoid transmission.

Interactions among Genetics and Environmental Factors

The occurrence of NCDs is the result of the interactions among genetics and environmental factors. Individuals with genetic defects who are then exposed to unfavorable environmental factors will be more susceptible to diseases. These diseases may occur at an early age and may be more serious. But if those who have genetic defects maintain reasonable healthy lifestyles and avoid exposure to environmental risk factors, they could probably avoid the diseases or have a better prognosis even after disease onset. For those who do not have genetic defects, if they are exposed to adverse environmental factors long-term, they are still susceptible to the disease.

PREVENTION STRATEGIES AND INITIATIVES

For the prevention and control of NCDs, comprehensive public health approaches targeting the human lifespan are required. Such interventions should target people in different groups. There are two types of interventions: population-wide interventions and individual health care interventions. Population-wide interventions and individual health care interventions are not completely separate. When combined, they may save millions of lives and considerably reduce the burden of NCDs.

Population-Wide Interventions

Although a number of risk factors are in the level of the so-called "normal range" for the general population, individuals still face risks for various NCDs. Thus, a population-wide intervention is necessary. This strategy refers to the appropriate health policies implemented by the government, including health education, health promotion and community intervention. It focuses on controlling the major risk factors in the whole population, preventing disease occurrence and reducing disease incidence and prevalence. Population-wide interventions act on the risks among the general population rather than determining which individuals are at risk. The population-wide intervention mainly focuses on the distal end of the causal chain, involving the common factors correlated with the root cause of many diseases. It can cover a wide range of people at a relatively lower cost. It is a compulsory way of protecting the health of the whole population.

Interventions to prevent NCDs on a population-wide basis are not only achievable but also cost effective. The best buys include:

- Protecting people from tobacco smoke and banning smoking in public places
- Warnings about the dangers of tobacco use
- Enforcing bans on tobacco advertising, promotion and sponsorship
- Raising taxes on tobacco
- Restricting access to retail alcohol
- Enforcing bans on alcohol advertising
- Raising taxes on alcohol
- Reducing salt intake and salt contents in food
- Replacing trans-fats with polyunsaturated fats in foods
- Promoting public awareness about diet and physical activity

In addition to best buys, other cost-effective and low-cost population-wide interventions that can reduce risk factors for NCDs include:

- Nicotine dependence treatment
- Promoting adequate breastfeeding and complementary feeding
- Enforcing drunk-driving laws
- Restrictions on the marketing of foods and beverages high in salt, fats and sugar, especially to children
- Food taxes and subsidies to promote healthy diets

Interventions with strong evidence but that currently lack cost-effectiveness research include:

- Healthy nutrition environments in schools
- Nutrition information and counseling by health care professionals
- National physical activity guidelines
- School-based physical activity programs for children
- Workplace programs for physical activity and healthy diets
- Community programs for physical activity and healthy diets
- Designing an environment to promote physical activity

Individual Health Care Interventions

In addition to population-wide strategies, interventions should also be undertaken for individuals who either already have NCDs or are at high risk of developing them. Evidence from high-income countries shows that such interventions can be very successful and are also usually cost-effective or low in cost. Compared with the population-wide interventions, individual health care interventions focus on the proximal causes of a disease. Health care interventions are easy to implement, and the effect is also clear, easily understood and accepted. However, these interventions have the limitation of producing a "labeling effect" on a person. Individuals who are labeled as "at high risk" may have greater psychological stress, resulting in anxiety or self-induced cognitive changes. In addition, this strategy focuses on individuals who are particularly vulnerable or exposed to specific risk factors. When the problems spread to the entire population, individuals who can be intervened are very limited, and this strategy cannot eliminate the core problem. Meanwhile, some scholars have also expressed concerns regarding the drug prevention strategy among the high risk individuals including how much the drug costs, side effects and long-term self-medication compliance, which will impact the effectiveness of this approach.

As in the population-wide interventions, there also are best buys and other cost-effective approaches in individual health care interventions:

- Counseling and drug therapy, including glycemic control for diabetes for people≥30 years old with a 10-year risk for fatal or nonfatal cardiovascular events≥30%

- Aspirin therapy for acute myocardial infarction
- Screening for cervical cancer, once, at age 40, followed by removal of any cancerous lesions discovered
- Early detection for breast cancer through biennial mammographic screening (50–70 years) and treatment at all stages
- Early detection of colorectal and oral cancers
- Treatment of persistent asthma with inhaled corticosteroids and beta-2 agonists

PREVENTIVE MEASURES

Prevention includes a wide range of activities, known as "interventions", which aim to reduce risks or threats to health. Primary, secondary and tertiary prevention are three terms used to map out the range of interventions available to health experts (Table 13-1).

Primary Prevention

Primary prevention aims to prevent disease or injury before it ever occurs. This is done by preventing exposure to hazards that cause disease or injury, altering unhealthy or unsafe behaviors that can lead to disease or injury, and increasing resistance to disease or injury. It is the fundamental measure to prevent disease and can finally eliminate the diseases.

Secondary Prevention

Secondary prevention, also known as the "three early" prevention, includes early detection, early diagnosis and early treatment of the disease. Secondary prevention aims to reduce the impact of a disease or injury that has already occurred. This is done by detecting and treating disease or injury as soon as possible to halt or slow its progress, encouraging personal strategies to prevent re-injury or recurrence, and implementing programs to return people to their original health and function to prevent long-term problems.

Tertiary Prevention

Tertiary prevention, also known as clinical prevention, is a measure implemented during the late stages of disease. Tertiary prevention aims to soften the impact of an ongoing illness or injury that has lasting effects. This is done by helping people manage long-term, often complex health problems and injuries (e.g., chronic diseases) in order to improve as much as possible their ability to function, quality of life and life expectancy.

NATIONAL AND GLOBAL PLAN

NCDs are now well-studied and understood, and this gives all countries an immediate advantage to take action.

Table 13-1 The levels of prevention.

	Primary prevention	Secondary prevention	Tertiary prevention
Definition	An intervention implemented before there is evidence of a disease or injury.	An intervention implemented after the occurrence of a disease but before it is symptomatic.	An intervention implemented after a disease or injury is established.
Intent	Reduce or eliminate causative risk factors.	Early detection, early diagnosis and early treatment	Prevent sequelae.
Examples	Legislation and enforcement to ban or control the use of hazardous products (e.g., asbestos) or to mandate safe and healthy practices (e.g., use of seatbelts and bike helmets); education about healthy and safe habits (e.g., eating well, exercising regularly, and not smoking); immunization against infectious diseases.	Regular exams and screening tests to detect diseases in their earliest stages (e.g., mammograms to detect breast cancer); daily, low-dose aspirin and/or diet and exercise programs to prevent further heart attacks or strokes; suitably modified work so injured or ill workers can return safely to their jobs.	Cardiac or stroke rehabilitation programs, chronic disease management programs (e.g., for diabetes, arthritis, depression, etc.); support groups that allow members to share strategies for living well; vocational rehabilitation programs to retrain workers for new jobs when they have recovered as much as possible.

National Health Plans

A national multisectoral action plan with national targets is a necessary framework for addressing NCDs and their risk factors through a public health approach. In 2015, 92% of countries reported that NCDs had been included in their national health plan. Of these, 64% had included NCDs in the national development agenda, 77% reported having a set of NCD indicators, and 60% had time-bound national targets. While 86% of countries reported having a national policy, strategy or action plan, only 62% reported having an operational integrated plan. However, trends in the availability of an operational integrated national policy, strategy or action plan are very encouraging, with a significant increase from 33% in 2010 to 63% in 2015. The most striking increase was observed in the African Region, with 73% of countries reporting having an operational integrated NCD policy, strategy or action plan in 2015 compared with 17% in 2010 and 37% in 2013.

Global Action Plan for The Prevention and Control of NCDs

A global action plan for the prevention and control of NCDs during 2013-2020 has been developed by the Secretariat of the World Health Assembly. For all countries, the cost of inaction far outweighs the cost of taking action on NCDs as recommended in this action plan. There are interventions for prevention and control of NCDs that are affordable for all countries and give a good return on investment. The total cost of implementing a combination of cost-effective population-wide and individual interventions, in terms of current health spending, amounts to 4% in low-income countries, 2% in lower middle-income countries and less than 1% in upper middle- and high-income countries. Continuing "business as usual" will result in loss of productivity and an escalation of health care costs in all countries.

In 2011, world leaders adopted a political declaration containing strong commitments to address the global burden of NCDs and gave several assignments to the WHO to help support country efforts. One of these was the development of the "WHO Global Action Plan for Prevention and Control of NCDs 2013–2020" (known as the Global NCD Action Plan). It has nine voluntary global targets and a global monitoring framework. The nine targets underscore the importance of prioritizing country action to reduce harmful alcohol use, physical inactivity, salt intake, tobacco use and hypertension; halt the rise of obesity and diabetes; and improve coverage of treatment for prevention of heart attacks and strokes and access to basic technologies and medicines.

Objectives of the global action plan

- To raise the priority of the prevention and control of NCDs in global, regional and national agendas and internationally agreed development goals through strengthened international cooperation and advocacy.
- To strengthen national capacity, leadership, governance, multisectoral action and partnerships to accelerate country responses for the prevention and control of NCDs.
- To reduce modifiable risk factors for NCDs and underlying social determinants through creation of health-promoting environments.
- To strengthen and orient health systems to address the prevention and control of NCDs and the underlying social determinants through people-centered primary health care and universal health coverage.
- To promote and support national capacity for high-quality research and development for the prevention and control of NCDs.
- To monitor the trends and determinants of NCDs and evaluate progress in their prevention and control.

Voluntary global targets

- **Global target 1:** A 25% relative reduction in the risk of premature mortality from cardiovascular diseases, cancer, diabetes or chronic respiratory diseases.
- **Global target 2:** At least 10% relative reduction in harmful alcohol use, as appropriate,

within the national context.

- **Global target 3:** A 10% relative reduction in the prevalence of insufficient physical activity.
- **Global target 4:** A 30% relative reduction in the mean population intake of salt/sodium.
- **Global target 5:** A 30% relative reduction in the prevalence of current tobacco use in persons over 15 years of age.
- **Global target 6:** A 25% relative reduction in the prevalence of elevated blood pressure or contain the prevalence of elevated blood pressure, according to national circumstances.
- **Global target 7:** Halt the rise in diabetes and obesity.
- **Global target 8:** At least 50% of eligible people receive drug therapy and counseling (including glycemic control) to prevent heart attacks and strokes.
- **Global target 9:** An 80% availability of affordable basic technologies and essential medicines, including generic medications, required to treat major noncommunicable diseases in both public and private facilities.

SUMMARY

Although the causes are complex, the vast majority of NCDs are caused by a small number of known and preventable risk factors, including tobacco smoking, lack of physical exercise and unhealthy diet.If these major risk factors are eliminated, approximately 1/3 of heart disease, stroke, and type 2 diabetes and 40% of cancer cases will be prevented. Numerous studies and long-term practical experience have shown that chronic disease prevention and control must be undertaken by the public health system. The primary, secondary and tertiary prevention principles should be combined together.

(Jianming Wang)

QUESTIONS

1. What are noncommunicable diseases?

2. What are the major types of noncommunicable diseases?
3. Intake of less than _____ grams salt per person per day is recommended by WHO.
4. Intake of less than _____ grams salt per adult per day is recommended by The Dietary Guidelines for Chinese Residents.
5. Human papillomavirus is related to _____ cancer.
6. What are the population-wide interventions and individual health care interventions?

IMPORTANT TERMINOLOGY

noncommunicable diseases	慢性非传染性疾病
risk factors	危险因素
population-wide interventions	全人群干预
individual health care interventions	个体干预
primary prevention	一级预防
secondary prevention	二级预防
tertiary prevention	三级预防
national health plans	全民健康计划

RECOMMENDED WEB SITES

www.who.int

REFERENCES

WHO. Assessing national capacity for the prevention and control of noncommunicable diseases: report of the 2015 global survey. 2016

WHO. Global status report on noncommunicable diseases 2010. 2010

WHO. Global status report on noncommunicable diseases 2014. 2014

WHO. Global action plan for the prevention and control of noncommunicable diseases 2013-2020. 2013

WHO. Global health risks: mortality and burden of disease attributable to selected major risks. 2009

WHO. Package of essential noncommunicable (PEN) disease interventions for primary health care in low-resource settings. 2010

WHO. World Cancer Report 2014. 2014

Index